THE NEW MILLENNIUM

DIET

START LOSING EXCESS BODY FAT
IMMEDIATELY

BY REVERSING
HABITUAL EATING SYNDROME

R.L. ERICKSON C.H.P.

This book is a work of fiction. Places, events, and situations in this story are purely fictional. Any resemblance to actual persons, living or dead, is coincidental.

ISBN: 1-4107-1034-3 (e-book)
ISBN: 1-4107-1035-1 (Paperback)
ISBN: 1-4107-1036-X (Hardcover)

Library of Congress Control Number: 2003090575

This book is printed on acid free paper.

Printed in the United States of America
Bloomington, IN

1stBooks - rev. 09/16/03

Acknowledgments

This research has evolved over the last 20 years. It started much as a mountain stream trickling between the rocks of immovable scientific theories. But just as the rock is slowly worn away by the stream's continual flow, so, too, do the misconceptions, false statements, and half-truths erode as new scientific evidence emerges, allowing new theories to supercede the old, and concluding that the body is chemically altering its fat storage mechanism due to socioeconomic stress.

I owe a debt of gratitude to the true pioneers of science. Though I will never meet these individuals, they and their work live on through their writings. Knowledge is therefore lost if not communicated to others. This book is an attempt to gather, build, and use past and present knowledge from generations of data to form new ideas that can be passed to the minds of people that can use the conclusions to better their life.

I would also like to acknowledge and thank the many and often unsung present ethical individuals of the scientific community, the men and women that take pen and pencil to the mountains of hardened theory and sculpt new and exciting conclusions, which helped in the preparation of this book to better humanity.

Finally, I would like to acknowledge my many clients and patients who opened their hearts and minds to me, that used the principles of this text to shed pounds of excess fat from their bodies.

Dedication

This book is dedicated to my late mother,

Nelma N. Erickson,

Table of Contents

SECTION TWO : Biology 101 Nutrients-body and mind

Disclaimer

This manual is designed to provide information in regard to the subject matter covered. It is sold with the understanding that the publisher and author are not liable for any misconception or misuse of information provided, as every effort has been made to make this book as complete and as accurate as possible. The purpose of this book is to educate. The author and/or publisher shall have neither liability, nor responsibility to any person or entity with respects to any loss, damage, or injury caused by the information contained in this book. The information presented is not intended to replace or substitute for medical counseling.

Prologue

"It is not the 'fat in' nor 'type of' foods we eat that is causing our current global weight gain phenomenon People today are overeating from a combination of factors that has created a synergistic effect, which in turn is altering our body's fat storage mechanism."

This book is a start to all other diets or nutrition plans. I ask that you please clear your mind of all past thoughts concerning information about *fats in foods*, *fad diets*, *strenuous exercise*, *weight control*, and *heredity*, and begin to learn how to properly control your urges to overeat, and start losing excess body fat *immediately* while:

- Eating the foods you enjoy

- Understanding how and why you store fat

- Keeping your *"metabolic lowering" starvation response mechanism* switched "off"

- Keeping your *"muscle burning" conservation gene* dormant

- Reversing *Habitual Eating Syndrome*

This text has gathered, prepared, and calculated; the history, cause and effects, charts, menus, and your revolving daily step rate calorie program for you. This text will help you understand that modern man is overeating from: *socioeconomic stress,* and by the addictive eating habits that we form as the culinary industry continues to biochemically engineer foodstuffs to enhance *taste, texture,* and *smell* You can start losing excess body fat *immediately* in just *two steps:*

1. Learning methods to lower your daily internal stress levels.

2. Follow the individualized *Revolving Daily Step Rate Calorie* program.

xiii

You are probably asking yourself, if this program is so simple and really works immediately, why haven't there been hundreds of books written on the subject? Why is this not the standard health guide?

These are valid questions – I asked them myself. The simple answer is MONEY!

Americans spend over $33 billion dollars annually on Weight control. Most diet books sell products. *The New Millennium Diet,* sells:

- <u>NO</u> prescription medication, medical device, or procedure

- <u>NO</u> exercise machines

- <u>NO</u> package of videotapes

- <u>NO</u> prepackaged special foods

- <u>NO</u> one-on-one 24 hour phone bank

- <u>NO</u> daily supplement powders, bars or tablets.

- <u>NO</u> "miracle" herb, vitamin, mineral, or special formula

<u>As long as the public buys into misinformation and half-truths, it is just not worth a large corporation's time for the royalty on one book and an Audio CD when billions can be made from expensive devices, procedures, or repeat supplement sales.</u>

Introduction

Have you tried different *restrictive food* or *crash diets*, only to gain back more weight than when you started? Have you become confused by authority misinformation concerning heredity and the continued belief that it takes strenuous exercise to lose weight? Are you convinced that a cure-all "weight loss pill" is just around the corner? Do you continue eating even when you are not even hungry?

Every diet book, Internet site, advertisement, healthcare agency, and fad weight loss program tries to convince you that the types of foods we consume, especially fatty foods, are the enemy, and by taking their pill, food supplement, prescription, or using their device, medical procedure, or buying their video tapes weight loss is assured.

Take a moment!! Food does <u>not</u> cause you to overeat. Food is really <u>not</u> the problem.

Food after all, is simply a transport mechanism for supplying the raw materials of life – *water, vitamins, minerals, proteins, carbohydrates, lipids* (fat), and *the energy* (calories) to sustain it. Food should therefore never be a substitute for one or more of the following: *love, companionship, friendship, power, addictive indulgence, or for emotional protection.*

Eating for these and the following reasons: *boredom, urge, reward, sweet tooth, security, or when you are not even hungry* is emotional and is actually caused by the continual flow of excessive stress hormones.

The United States Surgeon General and various national and international health agencies concur that over the last 30 years we have seen a worldwide obesity epidemic, even though per capita fat consumption has actually declined. Since this disease knows no social, economic, or racial boundaries, it is currently the second leading preventable cause of death in the United States, and according to leading health experts, will surpass tobacco use by 2007.

This text does not; however, intend as most diet books do, to worry the reader about food's so-called harmful substances like cholesterol, triglyceride, proteins, saturated fats, trans-fats, and carbohydrates, which have the potential to cause certain civilized diseases such as high blood pressure, heart disease, type 2 diabetes, gout, arthritis, asthma, or cancer. We will state studies and let you draw your own conclusions. The medical concerns of foods are then best left to discussions with your physician. This text is designed to be:

1. **A beginning** that does <u>not</u> restrict the kinds of foods you may consume or use the typical *"calories in, calories out"* philosophy. Understanding why you are overeating is the first step

2. **Enjoyable**. As you eat the right amounts of your favorite foods each day, you will lose excess body fat weight without triggering the "metabolic lowering" *starvation response mechanism* or experiencing the "muscle burning" *conservation gene.*

3. **Simplistic**. All the calculations contained herein are to assist you in determining your daily food intake.

4. **Knowledgeable.** *Excess body fat is the problem*, not how much you weigh or the fat content of foods. You will learn how the body responds to socioeconomic lifestyle changes, misinformation, altered engineered foods, and exhaustive stress apathy, and how to lose excess body fat while controlling the stressors in your life.

5. **A guide to relaxation**. You can reduce the continual flow of stress hormones causing *Habitual Eating Syndrome* and your weight gain naturally through a technique called guided imagery relaxation. The author's relaxation CD will allow the release of calming hormones that counteract and reduce stress.

6. **Safe low-impact resistance exercise programs**. Most believe, from authority misinformation, that it takes strenuous cardiovascular exercise to lose weight. This type of exercise can be painful on joints, breathing, and limbs, is difficult to begin and maintain, and takes longer to accomplish your goal. There are more effective ways to exercise, which you will learn from this text, but it is not nessessary. Even with little activity, excess body fat loss will still occur.

7. **A guide to better health**. After reading this text consult and work with your physician as a team. Explain your concerns and always ask questions.

8. **A stepping-stone**. After reading this book:

   a. You decide to eat in a healthier manner———— *Great!*
   b. You start or increase your fitness routine——— *Great*!
   c. Your lifestyle remains the same, but you
      lose excess body fat – That's also————————— *Great!*

    This book is intended to educate the reader concerning the history and nutritional development of the body and its functions, calculate your personal daily Calorie consumption rate, and along with the authors Relaxation CD, allow you to lower your stress hormone levels that control the effects of *Habitual Eating Syndrome.*

SECTION ONE

Man's Growth and Synergy effects on Fat

R.L. Erickson C.H.P.

1

Habitual Eating Syndrome And The History of Man's Growth

R.L. Erickson C.H.P.

Habitual Eating Syndrome

BEFORE I developed this program, I used an elaborate set of complicated nutritional formulas, as do most personal trainers, weight lifting champions, and bodybuilders. I knew the importance of maintaining and conserving muscle while losing body fat. I accomplished this through the right amount of proteins, fats, carbohydrates, water, workout routines, steam and sauna baths, massage, and tons of supplementation (amino acids, vitamins, minerals, protein shakes, and thermogenic agents). Believe me when I say that I was really ready to find an easier, less expensive lifestyle.

My hobby was more like work. Between owning multiple fitness centers, seeing patients in my hypnotist practice, and preparing for contests, most of my waking hours were consumed. And for all those hours pumping iron, money spent on supplements, tanning oils, and flights to and from competitions, I received, over the years, tons of self-gratifying looks and "ahhhhs", and a whole wall of $20 trophies and plaques.

At the same time I noticed that a large percentage of my patients were in a pattern of weight gain that was directly influenced by a previous stress event. They substituted food for one or more of the following emotional protections: *a replacement for love, companionship, compulsion, friendship, power, or addictive indulgence, and ate* for these and the following reasons: *boredom, reward, or security,* they were eating even when not hungry and then felt guilt. As we explored their problems, it was evident their bodies were attempting to build a protective wall between themselves and the outside world.

I began to formulate a developmental hypothesis based on research in the mechanics of our body's fat storage processes and on the physiological and psychological responses to excess stress hormones. As the stress hormones were lowered with relaxation therapy, weight loss began to occur *immediately.* I began to explore this phenomenon with other practitioners and to apply the results to our biological evolution with respects to stress and its relationship to habit, emotion, and protection.

As a species we have proven to be very adaptable and have flourished, unlike most animals that would have experienced extinction contending with these rapid synergistic stress changes, but biological change occurs slowly within our individual bodies. Humans living today unfortunately are caught within what I perceive as an *adaptive time phase*.

To combat this adaptive phase we have developed what I call *Habitual Eating Syndrome. A* combination of "stressors" (any agent that causes stress) coupled with our various biological protective responses has created a synergistic effect altering man's entire *nutritionally balanced body fat storage mechanism. Synergy* is defined as an interaction of agents, actions, or conditions such that the total effect is greater than the sum of the individual parts.

Numerous synergetic stressors, especially in the last 30 years, have chemically activated a biological protective chain reaction:

1. The body over-produces stress hormones that the system has not had sufficient time to adapt or control.

2. This over-stimulated chemical reaction begins to alter the fat storage mechanism.

3. The body begins to build a "protection layer" of fat between it and the outside world.

4. *Habitual Eating Syndrome* (eating ever-increasing amounts of calories to build and maintain this protective layer)

Fat is our body's protective response mechanism. Numerous physical and socioeconomic stressors have Modern Man accumulating excess body fat today not as "energy storage" for future famine, as a "shock absorber" for actual physical trauma, or as "insulation" for extreme temperature variants, as was the case for our prehistoric ancestors, but as "protection" against perceived, imaginary, and/or real stress events.

The conclusion: *Habitual Eating Syndrome* is the effect of this altered protective response mechanism, which increases appetite while lowering your basal metabolic rate (BMR) causing you to eat for reasons other that survival by consuming extra calories that build and maintain a "protection layer" of fat against perceived, imaginary, or actual stressors.

To determine if you have *Habitual Eating Syndrome*, I have complied the following questionnaire:

Habitual Eating Syndrome Questionnaire

1. Do you eat or drink when you are bored?
   Yes___ No___

2. Do you sometimes imagine food as a friend or companion?
   Yes___ No___

3. Do you use food as a reward?
   Yes___ No___

4. Were you taught as a child to eat everything on your plate?
   Yes___ No___

5. Do you often wake feeling hungry?
   Yes___ No___

6. Do you eat when you are not hungry?
   Yes___ No___

7. Do you eat more when you are emotional or stressed?
   Yes___ No___

8. Do you often snack after meals?
   Yes___ No___

9. Do you buy food in bulk to save money?
   Yes___ No___

10. Do you feel guilty after overeating a meal or snack?
    Yes___ No___

If you answered, "yes" to four or more of these questions, you have *Habitual Eating Syndrome*. These questions are designed to help you understand that you are overeating for emotional not biological reasons. This understanding is the first step in losing excess body fat weight.

World Population Growth

Although man's evolutionary path dates back millions of years, archeological evidence suggests that modern man first appeared about 200,000 years ago. It took 190,000 years (approximately 10,000 years ago) for world population to reach one million (The size of greater Indianapolis Indiana.) About this time a worldwide shift from hunter-gather to an agricultural based society emerged, and the first evidence of bioengineering food was documented. At 8,000 years ago the population had grown five fold, and by the construction of the Egyptian pyramids 5,000 years ago, world population had reached seven to ten million (the size of New York City). It was at this point that population began to grow geometrically. At the BC/AD timeline population was estimated at 250 -300 million. Population growth reached one billion in 1800, — two billion in 1930, —— three billion in 1960, — six billion in 1990. It is currently estimated that by 2060— ten billion (10,000,000,000) people will inhabit planet Earth.

Nutritional Growth: Bioengineering Begins

For over 95 percent of our existence on this planet modern man has been classified as hunter-gatherers; however, Man's lineage to nutritional evolution dates back million of years. During this seemingly unfathomable time–span, wild game, fish, fowl, vegetables, tubers, fruits, fibers, grasses, herbs, nuts, and seeds, plus the plants that produced them, all contributed to prehistoric man's nutritional cornucopia. Man thus evolved by eating all types of food groups, even so-called fatty foods.

As hunter-gatherers prehistoric man could only forage within a defined geographical area, usually within just a few miles, because he did not want to expend more energy hunting food than the energy in the foods he ate. Fortunately, grains and wild creatures were so abundant that prehistoric peoples needed only to consume grains like barley, flax, and corn as meal or gruel and/or to migrate and hunt great food herd animals.

With population growth came increased food demands. Wild game and grains became harder to find, and new methods for food production emerged. Man needed foodstuffs that could be stored easily over long periods of time, and with little spoilage.

Archeological evidence on two separate continents confirms that approximately 10,000 years ago man began to bioengineer grains, mainly wheat and corn, into hybrids that could produce flour. Flour was higher in calories, easier to transport and store, and had less spoilage. Similar crossbreeding techniques were then used for the domestication of certain animals. These new breeds became more energy efficient as their calorie content (fat and protein percentage) increased over that of their wild ancestors.

Farming and livestock soon caused small tribal bands to give way to towns and cities; merchants and farmers replaced hunters and gatherers. Man, no longer held by geographical boundaries, began to barter, exporting and importing foods from other lands thousands of miles away.

Whole populations began eating engineered foods and foods that were foreign to them. Breads from corn and wheat thus played an especially vital role in the development of human civilization. In geologic time, we changed our nutritional habits in a blink of an eye.

Scientific evidence also indicates that the occurrence of certain so-called civilized diseases, high blood pressure, heart attack, mental disorders, obesity, diabetes, gout, and cancer started to rise dramatically at about this same period

High calorie, low fiber engineered foods are thought to be the leading cause of these so-called civilized diseases. Engineered and many foreign foods were easier for the human body, which is chemically slow to adjust, to digest. These new high calorie, low fiber foods were also being consumed in ever-higher ratios to native foods, increasing weight, gout, cancer and diabetes problems.

Stress also played a major role as man was forced into close contact with other people. Migration to new farming sites, towns and city planning, laws, religious mandates, new modes of transportation, political strife, and family matters all created new stressors, which influenced man's everyday world.

Evolution generally occurs over long time periods. The body hasn't had enough time to adjust to these fast paced stressors and internal chemical alterations. Today's stressors and alterations are compounding at speeds the body can't handle, wreaking havoc with the body's protective fat storage mechanism.

Most foodstuffs we eat today are chemically engineered or altered in some form—trans-fatty acids, sugar substitutes, carbonated water, food coloring, genetic changes in fruits, vegetables, and fowl, steroid meats—the list is endless

Food labels today, most of which even a scientist cannot decipher, contain such garble it is little wonder that we and our bodies have trouble distinguishing good from bad. Couple today's increasing stressors with engineered foods, designer prescription medications, and lack of physical activity, and one begins to understand the tremendous strain our body is forced to endure. It is little wonder that a vast and increasing portion of the population uses body fat as protection from depression, abuse, pain, anger, and hurt.

Note: *We are so out of control with this insistent drive for food consumption that the creation of a whole food industry just to satisfy our munchies and snack cravings has emerged with foods containing little to no nutritional value.*

Social Growth: Food Shapes Our Civilization

Man did not evolve or posses super-sensitive sight, hearing, taste, or smell, nor the survival tools of fangs, claws, speed, strength, or a tough hide. To survive, man had to evolve a brain (see The Brain and Nutrition) that could out-think his opponent. Our biological appearance, internal structures and stress response mechanism, in a large part, owe their existence to the types of and ways in which our very early prehistoric ancestors hunted and gathered food. This continually adaptive process is a major contributing factor in the biological and psychological responses of modern man.

Prehistoric man evolved a stress response mechanism as his main defense. When confronted with physical events such as large animals, competing individuals, wars with other tribes, certain mating rituals, and climatic changes, the body would release certain stress hormones, giving it immediate extra strength for fighting or fleeing. This response mechanism, kept in check with extended periods of relaxation, was quite effective.

As man's knowledge and social skills advanced, population increased dramatically. Man as a hunter-gatherer, about 10,000 years ago, a mere tick of the clock in geologic time, began the transition to farmer and city dweller. Our stress response system was changing dramatically, as continued social growth added a new stress.

The formation of cities, towns, counties, states, kingdoms and parliamentary governments raised new social stressors: laws, religions, crowded conditions, economic pressures, social interaction and political hierarchy.

Social evolution had, up until this time, occurred gradually, as had our biological evolution, but in the last 5,000 years; social growth has accelerated beyond our capacity to physically adjust.

Social growth and population increased with the advent of metallurgy (copper, bronze, steel,), then by machines, computers and robotics. Many great civilizations and later world economies rose, only to be replaced by other nations, as witnessed by the Greek, Egyptian, Assyrian, Aztec, Zulu and Chinese dynasties, the Roman Empires, Dark Ages, Renaissance Period, Age of Enlightenment, the Industrial Revolution, and modern technology, leading to today's advanced computer age.

As man struggled with increasingly new stressors, great wars raged and were extinguished, civilizations rose and fell, and in the last 30 years socioeconomic growth has been especially damaging with the advances in instant media attention, corporate wealth, continued population growth, and apathy adding to ever increasing stressors. These stressors have had an adverse affect on our fat storage mechanisms.

Today's Social and Individual Views of Weight Control

Social Views:

Just as Stress is our body's defense mechanism, Fat is our body's protective response mechanism.

According to the Centers for Disease Control (CDC), 64 percent of U.S. adults are overweight or obese. *Excess body fat* accounts for more than 300,000 preventable deaths each year in the United States, second only to deaths related to smoking.

It is estimated that this number will surpass smoking related deaths within the next five years. Obesity has been termed an *epidemic* and established as a *disease* by the United States Surgeon General.

Obesity among adults has nearly doubled since 1980. This dramatic increase in excess body fat started in the 1970s with:

- The 1977 Senate's Select Committee on Nutrition and Human Needs when it issued its dietary guidelines. In their report, a *War on Fats in Foods* was declared as fat was acknowledged as having the equivalent danger to cigarette smoking.

- The Food Pyramid, a plan showing what proportions and types of foods to eat each day, was introduced at about this same time, and in my opinion and that of others within the medical and scientific communities, was misused and misinterpreted.

- A study released by a well-known institute contending that moderate to strenuous cardiovascular exercise is the best conditioning and fat loss fitness routine.

Federal and state government adopted these three forums, and today, twenty-five years later, they are still enforced. To counteract this rise in excess body weight, a *War on Fats in Foods* was declared. Since fat has twice the calories as protein or carbohydrates, this was seen as a logical solution. As a result, a surge in increased amounts of carbohydrates and sugars replaced fats in an attempt to lower calories.

Unfortunately, the opposite occurred, as people equated _no fat_ with _no calories_, and stress eating continued to increase the per capita caloric intake. Presently low-fat/no-fat foods have been found to actually have only a few calories less than their traditional fat containing predecessors. Since low- to no-fat foods lack the **satiety**

factor, the satisfying fullness that fat in foods produces, stress eaters consume greater quantities.

Also in the early 1980s focused attention also began on a more leisurely "at home" lifestyle. With the new debate raging on so-called good and bad foods and a glut of movie star aerobic exercise gurus, new multi-billion dollar industries in fad diets, home exercise equipment, food supplements, videotapes, mass misleading advertising, prescription obesity drugs, medical devices, and procedures emerged. People paid, but obesity numbers continued to skyrocket.

Within the last ten years alone, the estimate for calorie consumption, according to an international United Nations study for persons living in the United States has grown from 3,250 to 3,650 Calories per day. Lower fast food costs and super-sizing portions are thought to be the leading factors, but they do not explain our craving to eat when not hungry or from habit. The *'War on Fats in Food'* is being lost because it is not the underlying problem.

Note: high carbohydrate and sugar fat replacements exhaust insulin supplies or cause cells to become insulin-resistant leading to diabetes, another disease that is growing at epidemic proportions, causing new social stressors.

Individual Views:

1. Individuals with excess body fat are more likely to develop stroke, heart disease, high blood pressure, diabetes, gallbladder disease, joint pain (gout), interrupted breathing during sleep (sleep apnea), and wearing away of the joints (osteoarthritis).

2. Our nation's population acknowledges these medical statistics but continues to consume ever-increasing numbers of calories

while lowering physical activity, thus storing excessively dangerous levels of body fat.

- Why? Because, we are eating today for reasons other than survival. It has become the dominant entertainment in our lives. The statement "we live to eat instead of eating to live" has never rung truer. Our nation's top pastime is fast becoming food. We have become social eaters due to the numerous socioeconomic stressors in our cultural lifestyles,

3. Who promotes these Problems? Those that gain wealth from misinformation, half-truths and political posturing, any industry, Internet site, or special interest group that has relied on a monetary food (no pun intended) chain of greed, emotions, or quick fixes, with the *guarantee* that a pill, procedure, or device will replace or cure our preventable medical problems. The human body, although plastic, has not had time to adapt to social changes. Excess body fat is our basic protection against perceived, imagined, and/or real socioeconomic stress.

4. Many sincere scientists, physicians and politicians want to help; however, the very industries that created the problems are the ones that they turn to for advice. With billions of dollars at stake, confusion, scare tactics, authority misinformation, and political correctness, our nation is accepting obesity the *epidemic*—the *disease*—as the norm. If this trend of overweight conditioning is allowed to continue, our future generations may eventually be in great peril.

2

Synergy

R.L. Erickson C.H.P.

Socioeconomic Mind/Body Reactions

In my college chemistry class, I was taught that synergy *was the cooperative action of agents, such that the total effect is greater than the sum of the effects taken independently.* Or two plus two can equal five.

In my opinion there are eight major synergistic socioeconomic elements that have contributed to excess stress creating *Habitual Eating Syndrome* and the resultant explosion in food consumption to promote the "protection layer" of excess body fat.

- Apathy / eating when stressed or bored

- Competition wealth at any cost

- Frivolous law suites and malpractice

- Instant media and authoritative misinformation

- Abundant and chemically altered food supplies

- Lack of physical activity

- Political correctness

- A magic "weight loss pill" is just around the corner

Anyone of these agents could, in and of itself, be a formidable foe for the person struggling with a weight problem; but in combination and with the synergistic effects of the above-mentioned elements, the struggle can be enormous without the knowledge or tools to combat them.

We cannot change socioeconomic forces overnight. The monetary food chain is just too large. We can, however, start by breaking the first link. Restraints can be put in place at the personal level. You, as an individual, are the first link in the monetary food chain.

Apathy and Eating When Stressed or Bored

We are eating out of boredom and stress today at alarming rates. Civilization has developed complex social stressors and many new mental and emotional challenges, leading to new social *perceived, emotional, and imagined* future stressors.

Personal stressors include our personal involvement in war, enemies, natural disasters, illnesses, physical accidents, abuse, noise, the death of a loved one, divorce, personal financial problems, drug problems, children and or grandchildren, single parenting, affairs of the heart, personal fitness and health, burning toast, taking tests, hurt feelings, and low self-esteem or self-worth.

New social, *perceived emotional, and imagined* future stressors flood our thoughts with current upsetting occurrences that does not involve or affect us personally, yet are stressful. 'Telafriend' became telegraph, then telephone, and today television.

A growing number of people are experiencing phobias, fears, hatred, and hostility as they are bombarded with negative reports in newspapers, on the radio and television, in the movies, and on the Internet. Man's misfortunes are reported daily, in many cases just to increase ratings, concerning terrorists, famine, war, murders, mass transit collisions, severe weather damage, financial problems, and political opposition scare tactics of possible future doom for certain population groups. Imagined and emotional stressors have us literally feeding on negative news.

Regrets of past failures or stressful events, most never experienced, have started to control everyday life. *Today over 80% of individuals concentrate on past negative events that they have experienced, heard, or seen*, and then fear the future because these events may recur.

Stress-related illnesses. Many doctors estimate that stress is involved in more than half of all illnesses. Stress hormones that act on the heart, blood vessels, and lungs may contribute to heart disease, high blood pressure, and asthma. Prolonged elevation of blood sugar can influence development of diabetes. The stress response forces blood to leave the organs and move to muscles, leading to diseases of the stomach and intestines. Extended exposure to mental and emotional stressors can lead to difficulties sleeping, making decisions, depression, anger, and fear. Stress releases Glucocorticoid hormones (cortisol) that can interfere with the body's autoimmune system. During prolonged or repeated stress, people may find themselves more likely to get colds, flu, and many other diseases.

Stress is a main contributor for our food consumption and *to weight gain*. Negative habits and emotions cause the body to store subcutaneous fat to guard against perceived, imaginary, and real attacks. Apathy and increased body fat is the reward for our constant worry.

Competition Wealth at Any Cost

Within the last 30 years, businesses with a sole proprietor or owned by a partnership have given way to the torrid pace of the corporate structure, as household incomes and the subsequent wealth of industrialized nations flourished. Corporate formation in the 1990s hit all-time highs. More individuals entered the stock market and the 401k retirement programs were based on corporate performance.

Stress on the corporate hierarchy to achieve at any cost has left laws and moral codes shattered, along with the hopes and dreams of many Americans. *We are currently in a kind of mass depression and are buffering that depression with excess body fat.*

Today, for example, if just one type of procedure or device fails to meet certain expectations, billions of dollars can be lost around the world in the stock market. The competition between manufacturers is fierce. Stress, as shareholders hold the officers and board of directors accountable, often forces moral and social codes (false accounting practices, fraud, scandal, and stealing) to be broken.

This leads to false advertising, misinformation, half-truths and questionable selling techniques that have the consumer completely at the mercy of big corporate sponsors.

Frivolous Lawsuits and Malpractice

It is chic today to sue. Frivolous lawsuits are filed on behalf of individuals who do not want to take responsibility for their own actions usually seeking recognition or trying to make a quick dollar. Competing companies sue over various types of corporate law. Nations sue nations. This has caused insurance rates to skyrocket. It is easy to see that to *not offend anyone lest you be sued*, leads to continual stress on our society.

The rapid climb in medical lawsuits has pushed physician malpractice insurance premiums to all-time highs, forcing physicians to form *local standard medical protocols* that limit many good doctors from prescribing new medical procedures or new medications, lest they be sued. The high cost of malpractice insurance, often over $100,000 per year, is driving them out of private practice. Today, rather than treating patients in ways unique to the individuals they are dealing with, many physicians are reduced to just dispensing the standard prescriptions.

Abundant Food Outlets and Chemically Altered Foods

Although raw material costs have dropped significantly within the last five years as more land around the world is cleared for cultivation, trade agreement restraints are eased, and development of genetically engineered seeds accelerates growth, producing larger yields per acre, the per capita per day food supply in the Unites States has kept an amazingly close pace with population growth and has changed little since 1909.

According to the U.S. Department of Agriculture's Center for Nutrition Policy and Promotion, per capita daily Calorie supplies from 1909–19 were 3400 Calories and from 1990–99 they increased to 3700 calories. *The problem is we are eating more at near capacity, 3650 calories, per capita per day.* Why?

- Millions spent on altering engineered foods for taste, texture, smell, and consistency
- New advertising gimmicks aimed at children (mainly small toys)
- Innovations in packaging and food delivery
- Increasing food trade in what is generally called the *fast food market*
- Chemically altered foodstuffs and filler additives that produce ever larger overall portions
- Misleading claims that **no** fat means **no** calories.
- Socioeconomic stress

It is little wonder that man, eating for reasons other than survival, has created this overweight epidemic

Since 1991, there has been a surge in high-calorie fast food outlets providing inexpensive engineered foods. During this same time period, our consumption rate has increase by a daily average of over 400 calories. This is the annual average consumption of an additional

146,000 calories or the equivalent in additional annual body fat of 41.7 pounds per year; evidenced by the fact that 64% of the population is overweight. *Yet overall **fat consumption** during this same time period has decreased.*

High fat content in fast food establishments is a problem. However, obviously with fat consumption decreasing, our appetite for greater consumption allows these operations to flourish. A combination of factors exist today that is forcing us build a protective fat layer: modern conveniences, making it possible to do much less work, growing stressors, apathy concerning our physical appearance, and among the most lethal, a chemically altered food by-product trans fatty acid.

Trans fatty acid is a by-product of a chemical process called hydrogenation, and just may be the single worst altered food by-product ever created.

Oils (mainly vegetable) and mono- and polyunsaturated fat have a rather high spoilage rate and are harder to transport than solid saturated fat. In 1910, it was discovered, that by adding hydrogen molecules to natural unsaturated oils, a new chemically altered fat would be produced that was more solid at room temperature, could be transported and stored more easily, and had a lower spoilage rate. This method was little used, however, until the 1950s, when the popularity of the method increased as storage, transportation, spoilage and consumption demands mounted.

Unfortunately, this process yields a by-product called *trans fatty acid*. This altered fatty acid is chemically similar to essential fatty acids and can replace them in the liver. The liver uses essential fatty acids in the metabolism of certain amino acids, cholesterol, and other precursors to hormones and enzymes. The mimicking effect of trans-fatty acids has increased the potential for life-threatening diseases.

According to Mary G. Enig, Ph.D., F.A.C.N., trans fatty acids have been shown to:

- Lower the "good" HDL cholesterol
- Raise the LDL, the "bad" cholesterol
- Raise heart attack lipoproteins
- Raise total serum cholesterol levels 20-30 mg
- Lower the amount of cream (volume) in milk in lactating females and correlates with low birth weight in infants
- Increase blood insulin levels, increasing risk for diabetes
- Affect immune response by lowering efficiency
- Decrease levels of testosterone and interfere with gestation in females
- Decrease the response of red blood cells to insulin
- Inhibit the function of membrane-related enzymes
- Cause adverse alterations in the activities of the important enzyme system that metabolizes chemical carcinogens and drugs (medications)
- Cause alterations in the physiological properties of biological membranes, including measurements of membrane transport and membrane fluidity
- Cause alterations in adipose cell size, cell number, lipid class, and fatty acid composition
- Adversely interact with conversion of plant omega-3 fatty acids to elongated omega-3 tissue fatty acids
- Escalate adverse effects of essential fatty acid deficiency and the potential increase of free-radical formation.

This by-product of chemically engineered food may cause more deaths than all the combined wars ever fought – all because of greed, half-truths, and continued misinformation.

Unfortunately we cannot avoid trans fatty acids. They are now in almost every man-made food product we eat. We can, however, somewhat counteract its effects by incorporating naturally occurring essential fatty acids into our nutrition plan.

Lack of Physical Activity

From prehistoric times to the present, for over 95 percent of our existence on this planet, man has been a hunter-gatherer. Our skeletal muscles evolved as a necessity for finding and subduing food. The skeletal muscles were designed for everyday use, and even with today's modern conveniences, the majority of calories burned by our body are still through our skeletal muscles.

Our muscles are instrumental in our survival. The leg muscles, the body's largest muscle group, for example contract during walking or running, not only burning calories, but forcing blood up and back to the heart, leading many scientists to refer to the legs as our second heart. The leg muscles are so important to the heart that prolonged sitting, as on a long plane flight, can cause death.

Sixty four percent of our nation is now overweight. Socioeconomic stress, apathy, and emotional depression have increased our eating habits and changed our physical appearance.

A fitness center or health club may help relieve stress, apathy, depression, and change physical appearance, by allowing exercise to replace the muscular and cardiovascular calorie expenditures our prehistoric ancestors used during the hunting and gathering of food and building of shelter, and by taking our mind off our daily stressors. Unfortunately, where exercise in concerned, most consider it a grueling, sweaty waste of time. Most also believe that only prolonged cardiovascular exercise will work, again, by the following misinformation:

- A nationally recognized institute's study on cardiovascular aerobic exercise (in the 1970s) was adopted by the federal government and many state health organizations.

- The main health risk in the United States is heart disease. So, the cure-all is (as the name implies) cardiovascular exercise

- On average, more calories per hour are burned during cardiovascular exercise than from other form of exercise.

- Authority misinformation, slick sales gimmicks, and healthcare providers issuing prescription weight loss medications have us convinced that *weight is our problem,* touting "mortality charts" as our ideal weight.

- Most importantly a multi-billion dollar industry in cardiovascular exercise has grown over this last 30-year period, offering tapes, videos, fad routines, devices, and high-end computerized equipment.

The effect of this propaganda has been devastating to the majority of overweight people who often give up because of pain, strain and stress on joints, poor results, frustration, and time.

The good news: overweight people can start an exercise routine that is much more effective if they consider changing to *low impact resistance training.* Resistance training stimulates muscle growth by slowly increasing resistance using weight-bearing exercises. As the skeletal muscles increase and fat stores decrease from an increased exercise program, the muscle-to-fat ratio rises. By replacing muscle for fat on the body, a person will burn an ever-increasing number of calories, even at rest or while sleeping.

Note: For every pound of fat you replace with a pound of new muscle on your body, your body will burn 15 additional calories per day, everyday. Let me repeat that: *For every pound of fat you replace with a pound of new muscle on your body, your body will burn 15 additional calories per day, everyday.*

Think of *low impact resistance training* as depositing money in the bank with compounding interest. The more lean tissue (muscle) you have, the more body fat you will shed, even at night while you sleep.

For example, say two women, Ann and Beth, weigh exactly 200 pounds each. Ann has 110 pounds of lean tissue (muscle) and 90 pounds of fat, equaling 200 pounds. Beth has 125 pounds of lean muscle and 75 pounds of fat, equaling 200 pounds. If both women did exactly the same work, ate the same foods, slept the same hours, with no difference in lifestyle, Beth, because of her higher muscle-to-fat ratio, would burn an extra 225 calories (15 calories x 15 pounds) per day more than Ann everyday, day in, day out. Over a one-year period Beth would burn 82,125 more calories than Ann, or the equivalent of 23.5 pounds of fat.

If that isn't tantalizing enough, consider the fact that muscle is six times denser than fat, <u>not</u> heavier, as most have been taught to believe, again by misinformation. Thus, muscle takes up less space. You will look and be leaner with muscle than body fat weight.

Political Correctness

As our population diversifies, greater importance is placed on how society perceives our actions. This has created a controlling new stressor called *political correctness*. Today, almost any statement can offend someone. Words are merely subjective reality, but as we attempt not to offend by scrutinizing every word spoken, stress increases. In writing this book, I had to look hard at using 'man' to identify our species as possibly offending females. The word 'political –correctness' has thus become offensive to this author. It implies that to be correct you must be political. To be political means one must choose a side or position. One must then choose the majority opinion to be correct, and then convince others that have the minority opinion that they are incorrect. This leads to opposition, which is political, setting the stage for tension and aggression, and the battle lines are drawn.

Using the word 'minority' may imply lesser, small, or insignificant. A shorter than average person is now referred to as vertically challenged, and a fat person is now overweight or obese.

(These two words can have negative connotations because they may represent that a person is actually larger than just fat.) Again, weight, not fat, is the main emphasis when in actuality; it is excessive body fat that causes health problems. Remember the old saying "sticks and stones." Words aren't the problem; it is all about control. The more one is made to feel insecure, ashamed, or out-of-the-loop, the more control you gain over that person. This, of course, is an added stressor.

Certain politicians and business people use political correctness to create ever-increasing tension among special interest groups within the overweight community. An industry has thus developed, which, at the expense of fat people, makes money by using empathy to play on emotions and fears.

The healthcare industry is already feeling the pressure. In recent years, an inordinate number of overweight people are developing "my thyroid condition."

The *effect* may not necessarily be the result of a specific *cause,* a basic rule of the scientific method that has been tainted.

With chemical testing or just based on physician observation, thyroid medications may be prescribed in ever increasing amounts. However, was the cause of the person's increase in weight a result of thyroid deficiency, or did the increase in weight cause the deficiency?

The fat person gets stuck with the bill and the possible harmful side effects of the medication they may not need because of this "chicken or the egg" approach to medicine. How many forced diets, obesity medications, stomach and gallbladder surgeries have been prescribed or removed needlessly because of political correctness?

Fashion has also played along with an increase in body size. The actual size of dresses and pants has increased, but the labels have remained the same. What used to be a size 18-20 is now a 14-16.

To relieve this added stressor, let us start to not be politically correct but be politically active, by helping establish better nutrition legislation.

The Cure to All Problems Is "A Pill"

Since the dawn of civilization, man has been in search of "magic elixirs" to cure ills, restore youth, and offer immortality. With the birth of the pharmaceutical industry in the 1950s, our society has been slowly lulled into a false sense of security while waiting for our 'pill". We have become dependant on physicians as dispensers of medication, believing that a miracle drug, "the magic fat loss pill", is just around the corner.

According to the CRS (Congressional Research Service), there are currently over 1,000 drugs in testing with over $26.4 billion a year involved in research.

The pharmaceutical companies have, of course, become one of the most profitable international industries. They continue to enjoy an annual growth rate of about 13%. Prescription prices also continue to increase, as larger companies absorb competition, and there is very little a patient can do when a product in demand has no available substitute. The pharmaceutical industry will thus remain very profitable, as many prescription prices have risen faster than the rate of inflation.

Pharmaceutical companies are now allowed to advertise prescription medications in the mass media and slant the ads toward the benefits not the side effects. Often people are seen playing, dancing, and singing in commercials while the announcer is proclaiming "the side effects of this —————— drug can be nausea, high blood pressure, cancer, sudden heart attack, or even death in rare cases."

The idea of a "quick-fix pill" to solve our entire medical woes has us believing that whatever problem we encounter can be fixed by medication.

Medications are needed. I take them, but do we need them to control our lives?

Note: *medications are prescribed because they are potentially lethal, as witnessed by my mother's death from a widely used blood thinner that is actually derived from rat poison.*

Instant Media Misinformation

Advertisers are pushing the limit with misinformation. In addition, studies show that neither health professionals nor the public have a clear understanding of what constitutes health fraud or quackery.

There are many false nutritional facts established by a tainted scientific method, which are filled with half-truths and misinterpretation of nutrition and food science. The danger of nutrition misinformation is that it may be used to increase food fads or health fraud. *The U.S. Surgeon General's Report on Nutrition and Health* defines food quackery as "the promotion for profit of special foods, products, processes, or appliances with false or misleading health or therapeutic claims."

Claims: One such claim that is without question false is that, "*Cholesterol is bad and eating foods high in cholesterol will lead to heart disease.*" Numerous books have been written on this subject, cholesterol clinics have sprung up around the country, and low cholesterol foods are touted as nutritional.

Cholesterol, however, is important to our survival and reproduction. Many verifiable studies conclude:

1. High blood cholesterol in inherited.

2. Cholesterol is actually an essential fatty acid.

3. Cholesterol makes up an important part of the membranes of each cell in the body.

4. Cholesterol is used by the liver to make *bile acids,* which aid digestion.

5. Cholesterol aids in the production of vitamin D and certain hormones, including sex hormones.

6. Cholesterol is especially needed for the production of myelin, the insulation around nerve fibers.

7. Physical exercise helps lower the LDL (so-called bad cholesterol). Cholesterol-lowering medications will lower overall blood cholesterol.

Eighty percent of the body's cholesterol is made in the liver. Although studies have shown that cholesterol medications, which act on liver function, can lower blood serum cholesterol, to date *NO study has shown that eating high cholesterol or fatty foods will significantly change your long-term cholesterol count.*

Testimonial misinformation: tricks thousands of people every year. False claims of huge weight loss by consuming a vitamin mix, laxative inducing prescription, fat blocker, or stomach filler, among others, have caused serious injury and even death.

Health fraud within the fitness equipment industry is another major misinformation contributor. Many popular movie stars are paid large sums or guaranteed royalties to endorse weight loss aerobic tapes, abdominal machines, *no-resistance* muscle building devices, rubber bands, and stretching equipment.

The *effect* of these new socioeconomic stressors on the body is the creation of an excessive subcutaneous "protection layer" of fat; the *cause* is **Habitual Eating Syndrome**.

R.L. Erickson C.H.P.

3

Fat: The Misunderstandings?

R.L. Erickson C.H.P.

The War On Fat

The war on fat consumption and the rise in obesity has been raging for some 35 years. It started with substandard studies concerning the body's fat metabolizing system, the fact that fat has twice the calories as carbohydrates or proteins and the inference of a direct fat-cholesterol-heart disease linkage.

A subsequent multi-billion dollar industry blossomed to fight fat consumption (and to make money) starting with the 1977 Senate's Select Committee on Nutrition and Human Needs, chaired by then Sen. George McGovern (D-S.D.), when it issued its dietary guidelines. In their report, *fat in foods* was acknowledged as having the equivalent danger to cigarette smoking.

These same guidelines have not changed in over 25 years, and are in force today. Interestingly, the Harvard School of Public Health has conducted several studies on diet and health; these studies tracked almost 300,000 Americans over 20 years. Their conclusions suggest that total fat consumption per capita has little to no relationship to heart disease risk; that monounsaturated fats like olive oil actually lower heart disease risk; and that saturated fats present about the same risk as eating carbohydrates. Other studies have shown that although cutting down on fats would *delay* 50,000 deaths a year, unlike cutting cigarettes that can add years to your life, cutting saturated fats from the diet would only prolong life expectancy by a few extra months. *Our real concerns, rather than worrying about fat content in foods should be concentrated on excess stored fat in our body and:*

- Why we are eating foods in alarmingly larger amounts

- How and why the body stores fat

- What man-made by-products are in our foods

Body Fat Distribution

Obesity is not a single disorder. A variety of methods and criteria have been used to diagnose the presence of obesity. *The excess quantity of body fat deposits, and not just total body weight, defines obesity.*

Many people have been taught to believe that all fat cells contained in your body have existed since birth, which in turn determines your size. *This is a myth.*

It is true, we are born with differing amounts of fat cells because of our genetic make-up. But these cells are only activated if we overeat. Even more alarming, if we continue to consume more calories than we expend, we can continue to create new fat cells over our entire lifetime. Once a fat cell is created it remains.

Ninety to ninety-nine percent of stored body fat is called triglyceride. The body can easily use this type of fatty acid for energy. This fat is stored in special cells called adipocytes that resemble and act like little storage sacks. Adipocytes can only store a certain amount of fat. Once these cells are full, new cells have to be created to continue storing excess fat.

Collectively these cells are called fat. The majority of this tissue is called white fat and serves three functions: temperature insulation, shock absorption, and energy storage. This is the fat we see when looking in the mirror. Brown fat is much less noticeable and mainly is used for heat release, which is why it is sometimes called the "good fat".

Fat is mainly stored as *subcutaneous* (directly under the skin) and *viscerally* (inner body, usually around the organs). Distribution of body fat is usually gender related. Men tend to store excess fat above the waist (apple shape), women below the waist (pear shape). As women age they also tend to store fat above the waist in greater amounts, as aging causes hormone imbalances.

A quick test to see if you are at risk to form upper body fat is to calculate the waist-to-hip ratio. Measure the your waist and divide it by the measure of your hips. Women are at risk if the ratio exceeds 0.85 and men if the ratio is 0.95.

Nutritionalists use, as a standard for body fat storage, the equivalent storage of one month. Therefore an average woman should have 18-24% body fat and male's 14-19% body fat. As we age past 50, this percentage moves up by 6-8%, primarily because calorie-burning muscles atrophy (waste-away) as we become less active.

Our fat storage mechanism is being altered with today's socioeconomic stressors. The average person today carries two to four months of excess stored body fat, as the continual release of stress hormones causes people to store excessive amounts of fat, for protection against perceived, imaginary, and real stress, as a protective buffer response. The result: *Habitual Eating Syndrome*

R.L. Erickson C.H.P.

SECTION TWO

Biology 101 Nutrients-body and mind

R.L. Erickson C.H.P.

4

Nutrients and Calories

R.L. Erickson C.H.P.

Nutrients

A *nutrient* is defined as something that promotes growth or nourishes and repairs natural loss during organic life.

Man's survival is based on six nutrients broken into three basic groups: **water, micronutrients** (vitamins and minerals), and **food** (proteins, carbohydrates, and lipids). The food group may contain all other nutrients and also contains calories that produce energy. When we consume more food than needed, the excess calories are either excreted or stored as body fat. Note: There are many subgroups of important nutrients found within these six natural major groups.

NOTE: The waste byproducts of our socioeconomic growth are contaminating the very environments in which we live. It is therefore important that the air we breathe and the liquids and foods we consume, which can absorb these harmful elements, are as free from pollutants as possible. Equally dangerous to our health are certain by-products of bio-engineered foods that may prove even more toxic than previously imagined.

Nutrients today have been changed by man's intervention:

- **Exotic Foods**: We import foods that are foreign our digestive system.

- **Chemical Engineering**: Virtually every processed canned, packaged, or prepared food produced today has been altered chemically. Excess salts, coloring, and preservatives

- **Pollution**: Plants and animals that may become our food source absorb pollutants from the air, water, and soil.

- **Substitution**: Non-essential man-made chemical by-products often mimic essential food elements and replace them, altering our internal system.

- **Creation of New Food Sources**: Certain sea animals and rare plants that were not accessible until now are harvested as new foods.

Macronutrients: Water and the Food Group

Water is, of course, essential and the most critical nutrient. About 65% of our body is water. We can live without other nutrients for several days or even weeks, but we cannot go without water for more than about one week. The body needs water to help promote energy and digestion, to carry away waste products and to regulate temperature control.

Much controversy has developed lately concerning the amount of water we need each day. About 2–2½ quarts per day was the norm, but this figure may be revised downward due to misinformation.

The Food Group is our transport mechanism for supplying the raw materials of life and the energy to sustain it. Foods contain the other nutrients – water, vitamins, and minerals – in varying amounts, but through digestion food breaks down to just these four components:

- **Amino acids** from proteins

- **Sugar** from carbohydrates

- **Fatty acids** from fats

- **Glycerol** from fats

Proteins: Next to water, protein is the most abundant material in the human body, and the most complex, consisting of carbon, hydrogen, oxygen, nitrogen, and occasionally sulphur.

Proteins are composed of *amino acids*, the building blocks of life. There are over 100,000 proteins produced in the body by these amino acids. Virtually every function involves some form of protein synthesis. Proteins serve as one of the body's main building materials for muscle, skin, organs, neurons, cartilage, blood, hair, hormones, and neurotransmitters. In addition, every cell is made from proteins and contains protein enzymes, which speed up chemical reactions. Cells could not function without these enzymes.

As stated above, proteins are large, complex molecules made up of smaller units called *amino acids.* To date, some 50 amino acids have been discovered, although only about 23 are known to promote production of proteins. The body can manufacture all but nine essential amino acids. These nine, because they cannot be manufactured in sufficient amounts, must come from food or supplementation.

The best sources of protein are cheese, eggs, fish, lean meat, and milk. These foods are called *complete proteins* because they contain adequate amounts of all the essential amino acids.

Rice, legumes, peas, nuts, and certain vegetables also supply protein, but are called *incomplete proteins* because they lack or have an inadequate amount of one or more of the essential amino acids. A combination of two incomplete proteins, however, can provide a complete protein as together may they fulfill the total amino acid requirement.

Carbohydrates include simple sugars, starch, glycogen, and cellulose (non-digestible fibers). Carbohydrates are mainly used as an energy source, and are composed of hydrogen, oxygen, and carbon.

Green plants produce sugars through a process called photosynthesis. The plant combines carbon atoms with water using light energy and releases the by-product oxygen.

Sugars not used by the plant for energy are stored as starch or used as the plant's bone structure by producing sugar fibers called cellulose.

Animals cannot produce sugars in this manner, so foods containing sugars must be eaten. Human by-products of sugar oxidation are urine and carbon dioxide.

Simple carbohydrates are called sugars. All sugars end in *ose*: sucr*ose,* dextr*ose, fruct*ose,* lact*ose, and* gluc*ose*. The simple sugars easiest for human consumption include glucose, fructose, and galactose. Sucrose, lactose, dextrose, and maltose are a combination of two of these three sugars (e.g. glucose + fructose = sucrose). These sugars need to be broken down by enzymes. (See "Note on allergic reactions" below)

Complex carbohydrates include *starch, cellulose,* and *glycogen.* A molecule of starch consists of hundreds, or even thousands, of sugar glucose molecules joined end to end.

Starch is the chief form of carbohydrate stored by plants. Starch occurs in such foods as beans, corn, potatoes, and wheat.

Molecules of cellulose and glycogen, like those of starch, consist of many glucose molecules. Cellulose makes up much of the cell walls of plants.

Glycogen, or *animal starch,* is the chief form of stored carbohydrate in animals.

Lipids divide into two categories: simple and complex. They are insoluble in water solutions and soluble in organic solvents. Lipids are important to humans for six major functions:

1. They serve as structural support for cell membranes.

48

2. They act as a shock absorber for the organs (visceral fat).

3. They Provide protection from climatic changes (subcutaneous fat).

4. Fat layers are storage for water.

5. They provide energy reserves.

6. Certain lipids and their derivatives serve as vitamins and hormones.

Like carbohydrates, lipids are made from hydrogen, oxygen, and carbon. The two chief components of lipids are fatty acids and glycerol (alcohol).

Simple lipids are fat and oil molecules. The liver is the major site of fatty acid synthesis, and can synthesize all but two fatty acids. These two are essential fatty acids, which are not produced by the body and are needed for many functions, but particularly for cell membrane building and repair. Good sources for these two essential fatty acids are oils from peanut, safflower, flax, fish and common supplement fatty acids capsules.

Note: The sources of essential fatty acids suggest that early man evolved eating large amounts of plants and fish for survival, and a healthy diet today may need to contain more fish and plant oils.

Excess fatty acids in the blood stream are often referred to as triglycerides (which supply 30–50% of the calories in today's average American diet). Triglycerides can be higher than normal from inherited genetics, abnormal or diseased live function, or overeating.

Types of Fatty Acids: Fatty acids consist of three forms: *saturated* (animal fat, butter, etc), *monounsaturated*, and *polyunsaturated* (oils). Studies are indicating that fats are essential for survival and many oils are now found to even enhance weight loss.

Compound lipids are more complex fatty acids such as phospholipids and glycolipids. Upon oxidation, they yield not only alcohol and fatty acids, but also other compounds and derived lipids such as steroids, cholesterol, vitamin D, estrogen, testosterone, and cortisol. These molecules enhance life and help determine sexuality.

Engineering Fats: Saturated fatty acid molecules contain more hydrogen atoms than other fatty acid molecules. The more hydrogen atoms present, the more solid fat becomes at room temperature.

Fat Energy: Fats have become the "bad boy" of healthy nutrition through propaganda and misinformation. A fat gram (.35 ounces) has twice the calories (9 per gram) as a carbohydrate or protein. This fact has, in the last 30 years, led many misinformed individuals to start a war on fat.

Note: Allergic reactions, some individuals genetically may lack particular enzymes needed to break down nutrients into their smallest usable parts. (e.g. glucose + fructose = sucrose) This may cause a person to have an allergic reaction to particular foods, as the body perceives the particles as a foreign harmful substance and overreacts. In sever cases, some food allergic reactions can be fatal. It is recommended that these individuals consult a physician and avoid foods that may cause an allergic reaction.

Vitamins

Vitamins are essential because they regulate chemical reactions as the body converts food into energy and tissues. There are 13 vitamins vital to man, and all can be found in varying foods.

Scientists have divided vitamins into two general groups, *fat-soluble vitamins* and *water-soluble vitamins.* The fat-soluble vitamins—vitamins A, D, E, and K—dissolve in fats. The vitamins of the B complex and vitamin C dissolve in water. Small amounts of these compounds are needed daily. The following is a list of some of their more important functions.

Fat Soluble Vitamins:

Vitamin A: Involved in vision, smell, hearing, taste, growth, bone development, cell differentiation, and reproduction. Food source: meats, eggs, liver, milk, cantaloupes, carrots, sweet potatoes, dark green, leafy vegetables, and deep yellow vegetables.

Vitamin D: Especially important in infancy and childhood for bone development. Regulates growth, hardening, and repair of bone growth and hardness of teeth. Food source: sunlight, fish-liver oils, fortified milk, and others foods.

Vitamin E: Chief activity in all cells and tissues is as an anti-oxidant (prevents oxygen from destroying many other compounds vital to digestion and metabolism of unsaturated fats), stimulates development and tone of skeletal, heart, and digestive tract muscles. Food source: seed oils, vegetable oils, wheat germ, whole grains, cauliflower and green, leafy vegetables such as cabbage, kale, and spinach.

Vitamin K: Co-enzyme in liver's synthesis of protein, factor for blood clotting, required for function of proteins in bone and kidney, conversion of glycogen to glucose in energy metabolism and respiration. Food source: cauliflower and green, leafy vegetables such as broccoli, cabbage, kale, and spinach.

Water Soluble Vitamins:

Vitamin B complex is a group of eight vitamins. Listed are just some of their functions:

- Necessary in the building and repairing of neurotransmitters, which allow nerve impulses to travel from one nerve cell to another, especially acetylcholine for muscle control.

- Converts protein into usable energy.

- Promotes production of bile salts and the burning of fats and fat-soluble vitamins.

- Necessary for immune function and cancer prevention.

- Improves immune function in elderly.

- Involved in synthesis of nucleic acid (DNA).

- Needed for normal functioning of intestinal tract.

- Aids in carbon dioxide transfer reactions and serves as energy carrier of ATP.

- Required to convert toxic homocysteine into the essential amino acid methionine.

Food sources: meats, fish, and eggs or fortified foods.

Vitamins C: Necessary for wound healing, aids in forming red blood cells, critical in formation of dentin layer during tooth development, and essential for converting two amino acids, Noradrenaline and Serotonin, to neurotransmitters. Food source: cantaloupe, citrus fruits, strawberries, and tomatoes.

Minerals

Unlike vitamins, carbohydrates, fats, and proteins, minerals are *inorganic compounds*—that is, living things do not create them, and the body does not break down minerals.

Plants obtain minerals from the water or soil, and animals get minerals from mineral soils, water, plants or plant-eating animals. We in turn obtain minerals from the water and food we consume or by supplementation.

There are two types of minerals: *essential minerals* and *trace elements*. Although named, both essential and trace *are essential* for a healthy body. Some functions are:

Essential Minerals:

Calcium: Essential to bone development, required for muscle contraction, essential for nerve conduction and blood clotting.

Chlorine: Regulates fluids, electrolyte and acid-base balance in body parts, and stomach acid.

Magnesium: Catalyst in several hundred reactions - required in almost all reactions involving carbohydrate, lipid, protein, and nucleic acid metabolism.

Phosphorus: Promotes bone growth and strong teeth; used in muscle functions and cell wall formation

Potassium: Regulates fluid, electrolyte, and acid-base balance in the body, catalyst of many reactions inside cells, especially proteins, important for release of energy, prevents sodium from entering cells and interfering with protein metabolism

Sodium: Regulates fluids, electrolyte, and acid-base balance, serves as the main extracellular ion, determines water balance.

Sulfur: Aids in enzyme, protein, and connective tissue synthesis and protects us against toxicity.

Trace Elements:

Chromium: Improves glucose intolerance, binds insulin to cells helping its action in allowing cells to take in glucose.

Cobalt: Maintains healthy function of brains and nervous system.

Copper: Necessary for the synthesis of white and red blood cells, important anti-oxidant role.

Fluorine: Protects teeth.

Iodine: Supports thyroid function through its presence in the thyroid hormone thyroxine stabilizes and controls virtually all biochemical reactions in the body.

Iron: Is a part of hemoglobin in red blood cells, activates vitamin A, necessary for DNA, RNA, collagen, and antibody synthesis, resistance to infection by yeasts, viruses, and bacteria.

Manganese: Essential to development and maintenance of healthy cartilage, ligaments, discs, joints, and bones; important for inner ear development and balance; enhances immune function by stimulating activity of natural killer cells.

Molybdenum: Helps to remove nitrogen waste from the body through the formation of uric acid, involved in fat metabolism and energy production.

Selenium: Protects liver from toxin and free radical damage, maintains normal liver function, protects against lack of oxygen, improving function of mitochondria.

Zinc: Necessary for vitamin A metabolism and night vision, plays important role in stabilizing membranes necessary for insulin's ability to function.

*NOTE: New essential trace minerals periodically are discovered. In 1980, studies concluded that the very toxic **arsenic** was essential in trace amounts for iron synthesis and body growth.*

What Is a Calorie?

According to <u>World Book Encyclopedia</u>, "A calorie is a measure of heat energy, which is the amount of energy required to raise the temperature of one gram of water one degree on the centigrade thermometer at sea level." A *nutritional Calorie* (what you find on the food label) is actually a kilocalorie; one kilocalorie equals 1,000 calories.

If a label states that a piece of bread contains 70 nutritional Calories that piece of bread actually has 70 kilocalories or 70,000 calories of heat energy.

These 70 nutritional Calories (70,000 calories of heat energy) in that piece of bread will, upon eating and digestion, release 70 Calories of energy into our body. All calories are then converted to work, heat energy, storage, and waste. If a person consumes more Calories than they need, the body will either store the excess as body fat or excrete it as waste, whichever takes less energy.

An article written by Paul Doherty in *Exploring Food Magazine* Vol. 14, no.4 (1990) states, "A single peanut contains 1880 calories? Those of you who know about food calories may be shocked by this figure. After all, an entire lunch doesn't contain 1800 food Calories. The explanation lies in the capital C. One food Calorie, spelled with a capital C, is 1000 times larger than one physicist's calorie, spelled with a small c. A peanut actually contains 1.8 food Calories."

To work off that 1.8-Calorie peanut a 155-lb. man would have to climb the equivalent of a four-story building. There is enough energy in a standard milkshake to lift a 200-lb. man over the Empire State Building. *I imagine you are realizing that the thousands of calories you eat each day aren't going to be used up just mowing the lawn, walking on a treadmill for 20 minutes or watching the TV.*

Nutritionists use Calorie to represent a kilocalorie because it is easier to remember, easier to say, and not so large a number. It is, however, a disservice to overweight people because it is misleading.

Note: people might think twice if they knew that the typical fast food meal they were about to eat contained over 1,000,000 calories.

All foods contain calories, however, all foods are not equal in calories. Proteins and carbohydrates have about 4½ calories per gram weight, while fats contain about 9 calories per gram weight.

This 2:1 ratio was exactly what opened the door to the bad rap given to fats. As you have learned, we need certain essential fats to live. The only really bad fats are man-made like trans fats. Interesting, isn't it?

The body, as stated, is active even when you are resting, and thus needs a certain number of calories each day just to keep the body at a content temperature and for general maintenance. This resting caloric requirement, as stated earlier, is called our basal metabolism.

Basal metabolic rates (BMR) vary according to gender, weight, height, and age. As a general rule, females use 11-12 Calories per pound of body weight and males 12-13 Calories per pound for males. According to the BMR charts, the more you weigh the higher your BMR. This can be confusing and misleading to an obese person that has large amounts of body fat, which takes only 5% of our daily energy to maintain.

Body fat is nothing more than stored energy, and therefore uses very few calories to maintain. Yet most weight BMI and BMR charts count total bodyweight – water, fat, muscle, and bone – as one large, all-encompassing number.

There are no compensating factors that allow these charts to determine muscle-, water-, or bone mass-to-fat ratios. *Consequently, an overweight person is, in some cases, literally eating thousands of extra calories each day needlessly.*

A calorie is a measure of heat energy and not a nutrient like proteins, carbohydrates, and fats, but these nutrients contain calories. Water, vitamins, and minerals are also nutrients, but do not contain calories.

Food is thus mainly just a transport tool that animals and some plants use to move energy from one organism to another. Food should therefore <u>not</u> to be looked upon as *loved, caressed, worshipped, as a friend or companion, or used as emotional protection.*

R.L. Erickson C.H.P.

5

The Body: An Eating Machine

R.L. Erickson C.H.P.

Body Function

Unlike most animal species, humans did not evolve or possess super-sensitive sight, hearing, taste, or smell, nor the survival tools of fangs, claws, speed, strength, or a tough hide. To survive, man had to evolve a brain (see The Brain and Nutrition) that could out-think his opponent.

As man gained an upright stance, his legs and arms strengthened, allowing him more stamina to walk, run, swim, climb, and fight. He developed hands with an opposable thumb to grasp weapons and later tools, binocular vision for hunting and judging distances, and the internal formation of fat to store energy for hard times, insulation against harsh atmospheric conditions, and protection of vital organs from collision and minor punctures.

Our outward body parts evolved mainly to help us find food. All Internal organs, in some form, help in digesting, transporting and exporting food waste through the body for survival and to allow for reproduction. The body, both externally and internally, is therefore in a constant state of organic motion and in continual need of fuel.

Body fat thus evolved to store energy for lean times, to allow this constant state of organic motion to continue. Organic motion defines life itself. Body fat is therefore essential to our survival. If the body is deprived of energy and reaches a state of internal equilibrium, life is extinguished—we die.

Conversely, too much of even something essential can cause death. Water is the most essential nutrient, but drownings occurs daily in the United States. Excess body fat can also cause death by creating an intolerable internal environment, a form of chemical drowning.

The Digestion Tract

The digestive tract is one continuous tube that runs from the mouth to the anus called the *alimentary canal*. The foods we eat are too complex for our body to use, so from the moment food enters the mouth it starts to be digested. Digestion is the process of making food absorbable by dissolving it and breaking it down into simpler chemical compounds, chiefly through the action of enzymes secreted into and along the alimentary canal.

Enzymes, molecules produced by the body to speed up digestion, attach themselves to food particles and help in breaking down food to a more manageable size. When enzymes have performed their task, they release and go to other tasks. The same enzyme molecule can perform millions of operations per minute. Enzymes that work on digestion are collectively called *digestive juices* and are produced not only in the alimentary canal, but also by the salivary glands, gallbladder, and pancreas

When digestion is completed:

- The PROTEIN in that dinner steak (that you loved) becomes amino acids and peptides,

- The CARBOHYDRATES in the baked potato (savored with each bite) become simple sugars, and

- The FAT in the butter (generously applied) becomes fatty acids and glycerol.

These food substances, once broken down, can then be absorbed into the bloodstream along with vitamins, minerals, and water that are generally called *the body nutrients*.

In the mouth, as stated above, digestion begins. Chewing is very important to digestion for two reasons. As the food is chewed, water within the food starts to be released and mixed with saliva, which contains the enzyme *ptyalin*. Ptyalin and free water help change some of the starches in the food to sugar. Also, chewed food allows the digestive juices to react faster and more easily with smaller particles. Upon swallowing, the new mixture passes through the esophagus, which gently rolls and kneads it until it reaches the stomach.

In the stomach, food is thoroughly washed with hydrochloric acid and digestive enzymes by a tumbling machine-like action and churning motion caused by the contraction of strong stomach muscles.

The chemicals contained in stomach digestion are called *gastric juice.* It contains mainly hydrochloric acid and the enzyme *pepsin.* This juice begins the digestion of protein foods such as meat, eggs, and milk.

Starches, sugars, and fats are not digested by the gastric juice in the stomach because they are already chemical compositions of simple acid and sugar base.

Note: If, as we are led to believe, protein foods should be eaten sparingly, why did the body evolve such a specialized organ as the stomach to digest mainly protein foods?

After a meal, some food remains in the stomach for two to five hours. But fats, sugar, and other small particles begin to empty almost immediately. Food that has been churned and partly digested is called *chyme.* Chyme passes from the stomach into the small intestine as a thick, whitish liquid.

In the small intestine, the digestive process is completed on the partially digested food by pancreatic and intestinal juice, and bile.

The pancreatic juice is produced by the pancreas and pours into the small intestine through a duct, or tube. The pancreatic juice contains the enzymes *trypsin, amylase,* and *lipase.* Trypsin breaks down the partly digested proteins; amylase changes starch into simple sugars; and lipase splits fats into fatty acids and glycerol.

The walls of the small intestine produce the intestinal juice. It has milder digestive effects than the pancreatic juice, but carries out similar a digestive function.

Bile is produced in the liver and stored in the gallbladder. Bile flows into the small intestine through the bile duct. Bile does not contain enzymes, but it does contain chemicals that help break down and absorb fats.

When the food is completely digested, particles are small enough to be absorbed by tiny blood and lymph vessels in the walls of the small intestine. It is then carried to the liver, where some food is stored, and then into the circulation system for nourishment of the body.

In the large intestine, almost no digestion occurs. The large intestine stores waste food products and absorbs water and small amounts of minerals. The waste materials that accumulate in the large intestine are roughage that cannot be digested in the body. Bacterial action produces the final waste product, the *feces,* which are eliminated from the body.

Body Metabolism

Micro-metabolism occurs at the cellular level. Food is transported around the body by the blood and absorbed by cells. Once food has been reduced by enzymes to its basic components, *proteins* into amino acids and peptides, *fats* into fatty acids and glycerol, and *carbohydrates* into simple sugars, particularly glucose, it can be used by the cells for building, repairing and as fuel.

Metabolism is the energy transfer of these smaller particles that occur in our tissues, with the by-product of cellular metabolism being heat, carbon dioxide, and water. Excess energy is stored as body fat or excreted.

Different cells require different amounts of energy: muscle cells use 60–65% of our daily energy, brain cells use approximately 25% and 8–10% is used for digesting the food we eat. That only leaves 5–7 % for all other functions, including the energy to maintain huge amounts of body fat.

Heat energy, a by-product of metabolism, helps keep our body warm and, when properly regulated by the hypothalamus (an portion of our inner brain), at a constant temperature. Excess heat energy is channeled out through the skin as we perspire. During strenuous activity or in hot outside atmospheric conditions, water and some oils stored in the subcutaneous fat are released through pores in our skin, creating sweat. As sweat evaporates on the skin, the body loses excess heat much as an air conditioner cools a room.

Metabolism has two phases:

Anabolism, or *constructive metabolism,* during which cells combine to form molecules to build and repair.

Catabolism, or *destructive metabolism,* during which cells break down molecules to obtain energy and release heat.

The body is more anabolic than catabolic within two hours of eating a meal. During this time, glucose (sugar) levels increase, and the pancreas responds by releasing the hormone insulin.

Insulin serves as a trigger for cells to begin anabolic activities. When the level of glucose is low the pancreas releases the hormone glucagon.

Glucagon signals the cells to conduct more catabolic processes. High amounts of sugar and triglycerides in the blood from overeating can eventually cause cells to become insulin resistant, thus resulting in a form of diabetes. There is a direct link, therefore, between excess body fat and diabetes.

Macro-metabolism refers to the whole body's metabolism. We refer to body metabolism as the amount of calories (heat energy) produced during micro-metabolism. When we consume more calories than we need, the excess is stored as fat or excreted. In heat energy, a pound of stored body fat contains about 3,500 Calories. Heat energy released in a resting state (no physical activity) is expressed as the basal metabolic rate (BMR).

Most formulas calculate BMR at 11–12 Calories per pound of weight for a female and 12–13 Calories per pound of weight for a male. This difference occurs because males usually contain more muscle mass than females. As a general rule, a 150-pound male would thus burn about 150 Calories more each day than a 150-pound female.

6

The Brain and Nutrition

R.L. Erickson C.H.P.

Evolution of The Brain

Relying on previous data, most scientists studying brain evolution concluded that the brain increased in size three-fold in the last 2–4 million years. Recent discovery of a much older human-like skull may push these dates back an additional 3–5 million years.

One hypothesis concerning brain evolution is: as the DNA molecule used up its cellular memory storage area, brains cells evolved to handle the load. Since the central nervous system (CNS) is connected to all parts of the body via nerves, natural selection dictated that one end of the CNS, the brain, would make an ideal storage area—a logical choice.

The brain, to date, is the most complicated and diverse biological structure yet discovered in our universe.

Paul MacLean, a pioneer of modern neuroscience, has defined three distinct evolutionary phases in the brain's development:

1. *Reptilian* (the brain stem and surrounding motor functions, the *unconscious* mind)—controls aggression and basic instincts.

2. *Paleomammalian* (the limbic system, the *subconscious* mind)—controls perception, emotions, long-term memory, habits, and the body's autonomic nervous system.

3. *Neomammalian* (the neocortex, the *conscious* mind)—controls cognitive analytical thinking and short-term working memory.

Each phase evolved to store increased knowledge needed for survival.

These systems interact and are controlled by a kind of seniority system. The oldest system will usually prevail if there is conflict between parts. This helps explain why emotions and habits overrule cognitive thinking and physical demands overrule both of the above. Here are a couple typical examples:

You are watching a movie thriller that involves mountain climbing. The scenery is beautiful, but you have a phobia of heights. Even though you are sitting at home in your favorite chair, you feel uneasy looking at the screen. The subconscious mind controlling phobias supercedes the cognitive spatial mind.

Or *you are enjoying a wonderful walk in the woods. Suddenly you feel the hair stand up on the back of your neck, as you recall seeing a bear attack on TV last year. Even though there isn't a bear within 100 miles, you feel uneasy and the woods are now a place to avoid.*

Since the brain controls body function, it is important that you learn how to control the brain. This can be achieved if you remember this basic seniority system principle. Later chapters will teach you how to control stress, the main reason for which we eat excessively today.

The Neocortex and Limbic System Brain Structures

Together, the brain and spinal cord make up the central nervous system. They are covered by three layers of membranes and bathed in a protective fluid that acts as a buffer to help prevent injury.

All parts of our brain are interactive. Though evolution has assigned different functions to the many lobes and structures of the brain, studies indicate that neurons in close proximity to an injury often migrate to the site and/or take over the work of the injured cells. Excess stored body fat today is primarily the combined effect on our body of the following two brain structures:

The neocortex has been sectioned into functional lobes according to brain grooves.

70

- Frontal – cognitive thinking thought learning memory

- Parietal – sensory touch, pain, movement

- Temporal – hearing responses

- Occipital – visual information

- Brain stem – autonomic responses

- Cerebellum – coordination

The neocortex allows the use of cognitive capabilities:

- Attention, thinking, evaluating, insight, abstraction, goal direction

- Creativity, generalization, choice, purpose, seeking, planning

- Judgment, introspection, programming, preference, learning

- Short-term work memory – recognition of precepts

These lobes act as a kind of secretary, storing information or routing it to various older internal brain parts for further analysis. When viewed from above, looking down at the brain, a large groove divides the brain into a right and left hemisphere.

The limbic system, this ancient set of structures, is responsible for the following behaviors:

- Basic survival

- Pain

- Pleasure

- Anger

- Fear

- Hunger

- Sexual behavior

- The autonomic nervous system

It includes the Thalamus, Hypothalamus, Hippocampus, Cingulate Cortex, Amygdala, and Septum.

Note: This structure is the leading cause of our weight gain. The limbic system is responding to outside pressures and perceiving imaginary dangers to which it responds by protecting or shielding the body in a lining of subcutaneous fat.

Our entire brain is interconnected, or wired together, in a network composed of approximately 100 billion neurons, which are the main communication cells, and about 1,000 billion (1 trillion) glial cells. Glial cells are like butlers and maids to the neurons, protecting, supporting, and helping.

All 1.1 trillion neuron and glial cells have identical genetic material and the same genes.

Neurons

At birth, a normal human has close to 200 billion neurons. (The same number of stars, some estimate, that are in our Milky Way galaxy) About half of this amount will be cannibalized during early infancy by more active neurons. The remaining 100 billion Neurons must work in order to survive, as dormant neurons will die.

Neurons are wired to each other through a maze of structures called dendrites and axons. Dendrites receive information and axons deliver information. A single neuron may have up to 10,000 dendrite-axon connections with other neurons at points called synapses.

The synapse (or gap) allows for an electrochemical response in the form of chemicals called neurotransmitters to either be released or received as communication. Currently scientists have discovered some 30 neurotransmitter chemicals, including: Serotonin, Dopamine, Epinephrine, Acetylcholine, and Norepinephrine.

Neurons are constantly chatting with each other chemically and form a humming sound from 40–60 Hz (cycles per second). Many scientists equate this constant communication between neurons with consciousness.

Collectively, however, not all neurons are chatting at the same time, so the overall net electrochemical wave changes. Total wavelength activity runs from as high as 60 Hz in REM sleep to as low as .5 Hz in a coma. Alertness usually is considered to fall within the 14–30 Hz range.

The functions of collectively active neurons in a normal brain include:

- Perception (how we view the world)

- Behavioral sequences (habits)

- Reflexes

- Instincts

- Emotions

- Thinking

- Imagination and other integrative activities.

The neurons also allow us to view the world through:

Senses:

- Olfaction (smell)

- Sight (vision)

- Touch

- Hearing (auditory)

- Taste (bitter, sour, sweet, and salty) – texture may also be a part of taste

- Pain (special cells react to sharp or dull pain)

Sensations:

- Hunger, love, lust, sex, anger, hate, and fear

- Territoriality or possessiveness

- Dominance and submissiveness

- Irritability

- Serenity, sociality, parenting, and family ties

- Growth of emotions

- Self-preservation and aggressiveness

Glial cells

For every neuron in the brain there are 10–50 helper cells collectively called Glia.

The major function of glial cells appears to be a "supportive" role much like a housemaid or butler. Several types of glial cells are found throughout the central nervous system.

In the brain, glial cells serve as myelin sheaths, which use cholesterol (a form of fatty acid) as insulation, wrapping around nerve fibers, allowing them to conduct information more rapidly and without interference.

Other types of glial cells in the brain:

- Regulate the composition of extracellular communication functions,

- Clean up brain debris,

- Guide developing neurons to the right places in the brain,

- Store extra energy for active neurons, and

- Store fluids to complement neurons in certain metabolic activities.

The brain, which is about 2% by weight of the adult human, as stated earlier, uses a whopping 25% of the of our daily energy output to carry out all of its functions, mainly due to its constant activity and inability to store energy.

The brain operates mainly on carbohydrates but can use ketones, a by-product of protein synthesis during food shortages. The brain, through perceptions, emotions, imagination, and habits, controls our thoughts concerning food, and is more responsible for our overweight condition than our body's need for nutrition. *Learning to control the brain's response mechanisms is a major step toward controlling Habitual Eating Syndrome.*

7

The Mind: Stress, Memory, Consciousness, Imagination

R.L. Erickson C.H.P.

Stress

Controlled stress can be good, as felt upon winning a tough race, catching that trophy fish, sinking a long put, or winning the lottery – that rush of excitement that raises your heart rate and breathing, that feeling of exhilaration.

Stress however mainly evolved as man's main defense response to possible immediate death. It was an emergency response system to real physical circumstances in prehistoric times. Stress was particularly useful for such actions as:

- Hunting large animals.

- Defending shelter

- Tribal war

- Mating

A stress reaction actually prepares the body to fight or flee a threat by supplying it with a burst of energy and shutting down normal body function pathways. Any *event*, *thought*, or *situation* that causes stress is called a ***stressor.***

Stress causes the release of epinephrine (adrenalin) and glucocorticoids (cortisol) into the blood system. These powerful hormones induce the following reactions:

- Increased heart rate and blood sugar levels

- Sweaty hands

- Skin tightness

- Increased blood pressure

79

- Blood thickening

- Slowed digestion and excretion

- Muscle tightness

- Pain receptor blockage

- Negative emotional increase (hate, rage, anger, fear, anxiety) as the body prepares to fight or run.

As civilization developed, some physical stressors remained, including war, bullies, natural disasters, illnesses, physical accidents, bodily abuses, and noise.

But as society became more complex, mental and emotional challenges increased and we began to develop social and imagined physical and psychological stressors.

The Body's Reaction to Stress

Canadian scientist Hans Selye noted, while studying the body's reaction to stressors and formulating what he called The *General Adaptation Syndrome,* "Without stress, there would be no life." The body needs a certain level of stress, but when extreme or continuous stress occurs, our body responds according to a set of systematic reactions:

Alarm reaction is the first phase of this syndrome. It occurs when a person first senses danger. An alarm reaction begins in the brain when a frightening experience activates an area called the *hypothalamus.* The hypothalamus then sends nerve signals to the *adrenal glands,* located on top of the kidneys.

These nerve signals stimulate the inner core of the adrenals to release the hormone *epinephrine,* which is also called *adrenalin.*

Adrenalin raises heart rate, breathing rate, blood pressure, and the amount of sugar in the blood. These effects increase alertness and deliver more blood, oxygen, and food to active muscles.

If danger persists, a stage second is activated:

Resistance follows the alarm reaction. During resistance, the body attempts to return to a state of balance. Breathing and heart rate decrease to normal levels.

But the hypothalamus sends a hormone signal to a nearby gland called the *pituitary.* The pituitary gland then releases *adrenocorticotropic hormone,* also called ACTH.

ACTH travels to the outer layer of the adrenal glands releasing hormones called *glucocorticoids (cortisol).* These hormones keep blood sugar high to provide extra energy.

If stress continues at high levels, the body enters the final stage:

Exhaustion In exhaustion, energy reserves are used up; extreme fatigue and an inability to resist new stressors appear. Long-term stress can lead to very deep depression, serious illness, premature death, and is the leading cause of *Habitual Eating Syndrome.*

Memory

In computer terminology, the brain would be considered a bio-electrochemical hard drive. Memory, consciousness, and imagination are the compartmental software.

According to John Ratey, M.D., Harvard professor, author of *A User's Guide To The Brain,* and co-author of *Shadow Syndromes,* humans have developed many different levels of memory.

Memory allows us to build on past experiences, both analytically and emotionally. Memory, however, is not perfect, and often misinformation can be remembered as truth and lead to many pitfalls. About ¼ of adults can be convinced by authority figures or trusted advisers through false memory that events or ideas that never happened did actually occur.

Many commercials today rely on false memory and half-truths to sell products. Many legends become truth through false memory.

Memory is formulated at various convergence zones, areas close to the place where a specific memory is first imprinted on the brain. The brain then simplifies and reconstructs reusable elements into complex memory patterns. These patterns are then stored in separate compartments of the brain until needed.

When looking at a tree, for example, you might store the color in one compartment of your brain, the texture, height, type, background, smell, date, time, and your emotions at that moment in other separate compartments.

Memory, therefore, is very complex, and can be distorted easily by losing some or all these components from injury, illness, or mental abuse, or by simply not pulling all the components together at the same time for an occasional review. The more repetitive the recollection, the easier the memory is to recall. This can be both positive and negative, depending on your emotional state and recollection of events.

Learning enables information to become memory and thus helps affect future learning. We thus build upon our learned memories: arithmetic to geometry to algebra to trigonometry to calculus is an example.

This same memory learning mechanism may have negative consequences as we learn how to lie, cheat, steal, and swindle, or solidify addiction with ever increasing thoughts of the feelings brought forth by drugs or certain foods. Thus, the more a learned trait is repeated, the more that trait, even if negative, is strengthened hence the phrase "once a liar always a liar."

Exercising the brain strengthens memory just as weight training strengthens muscles. Playing mental mind games, reading, writing poetry, playing a musical instrument, solving math problems, creating hypotheses, learning new words all help strengthen memory.

Working memory is short. It helps us do everyday tasks like remember a number long enough to dial it or find the route to a new business in the neighborhood.

Working memory also is the recall mechanism for long-term memory. It holds multiple long-term memories so they can be recalled in an instant for the task on which we may be working.

Working memory is sometimes referred to as the "Noise of consciousness". When trying to concentrate or focus, working memory may be carrying on business as usual. An example of this phenomenon might go like this:

You are listening to a friend recall a vacation. You are looking, listening, and at the same time you are thinking about dinner, the kids, work, what you might be wearing tomorrow, what time it is. You suddenly recall a similar situation: "I did that on vacation," "I have been there." As this noise grows, it can be deafening to the point where you hear your friend say, "Are you listening?" Whoops!

There are various types of memory that our mind can utilize.

- *Subjective memories* are events that we sense and then interpret through what we have previously learned. We thus form immediate opinions and throw up roadblocks. This may be why many people hate to talk about religion, politics, or diets at parties.

- *Explicit memory* encodes factual events – names, faces, and things – that become consciously accessible.

- *Implicit memory* is responsible for skills, habits, and sensitizing events. These memories are retained without conscious thought. Implicit memory is very inflexible and slow to develop. Most memory moves from explicit to implicit.

- *Episodic memory* is the ability to place facts or events in a time sequence, remembering past events or future anticipations. Example: Where were you on 9/11?

- *Semantic memory* allows for the generalization of facts, events, objects, and spatial knowledge. Jim, at the time, your best grade school friend becomes a boy. Lora, your first love, becomes that girl I once dated.

Other types of memory that have less bearing on stress eating include **sensory, motor, visuospatial,** and **language.**

Evolution of Consciousness

Until the 1990s, most scholars agreed that cognitive thought or consciousness began some 40,000 years ago. The evidence supporting this hypothesis are cave paintings found all over Europe, showing man's awareness of religious events or of leaving an obvious pictorial record for future generations. Today, however, there is growing evidence that consciousness may precede this time period by hundreds of thousands of years.

New evidence is growing of ancient civilizations and/or groups of people that may have become extinct due to some large catastrophe such as a tidal wave, sudden rise in sea level, glaciations, volcanic or earthquake activity, destroying almost every record of their existence.

Recent burial sites found in the Middle East have uncovered clues that certain 100,000+-year-old societies buried their dead with what some envision as ritualistic flower arrangements. Various flowering plant pollens were found alongside the skeletal remains.

Others say this may have been a vain attempt at covering the smell of the corpse as it decomposed. In either case, cognitive thought rather than instinct would have been needed.

Consciousness allows us to think, imagine, and work out our instincts for the betterment of mankind. It is when we allow our thoughts to turn inward, to become negative, to imagine no end to a problem that consciousness can become our undoing.

An animal eats when instinct allows it to feel hunger. Most animals will eat until they are full then stop (exceptions are domesticated animals that have been "bred" to continue feeding).

Man on the other hand eats for a variety of reasons other than hunger or survival including emotions, habits, past sensitizing events, boredom, pain, or power. Evolution thus dictates us to control our perceptions and emotions lest we develop harmful habits.

Conscious/Subconscious Tug-of-War

What we are psychologically is determined by our past learned and sensitizing events. We filter every sensation, word, sight, sound, emotion, thought, and memory through what we have experienced.

If I ask five people to give me an immediate response to the word *apple*, I may expect to get five different answers. How we perceive our world, how we fit into that world, and what future that world holds, when viewed through our past experiences, forms our behavior.

The French philosopher, René Descartes, came up with a philosophical quotation: "I think, therefore I am." This statement has created many debates over the last 400 years.

Today, most view this statement as meaning that the way we think controls how we feel. "I think I *am hungry,* therefore I am hungry." "I think I *am bored*, therefore I am bored." "I think I *am sick*, therefore I am sick."

This confirmation of thinking and feeling becomes even more entrenched in our minds when we physically speak these words. When the senses of sight, sound, touch, and speech are included with thought, a majority of brain parts is put into action.

This repetitive confirmation allows the brain to solidify your thinking pattern with added authority to the point that you can actually *think* yourself fatter. Thus *negative reactions can spawn negative conclusions.*

In respect to *Habitual Eating Syndrome*, the conscious, analytical, scientific, thinking mind (neocortex) and the more primitive, subconscious, habit-forming, emotional, reaction mind (limbic) interact both positively and negatively in what amounts to a power struggle tug-of-war.

You want to lose weight and have tried tens of diets only to regain it. You "think" the problem is a lack of *willpower*, so you try a different approach, but in reality it is much deeper than mere willpower.

The conscious, analytical, thinking mind cannot understand why you just can't eat less, because the conscious mind only sees two plus two equals four, blue and yellow equals green, sugar is sweet and lemon sour.

The subconscious mind, however, is more primitive. It simply reacts to what you tell it to do. The subconscious mind does not know right from wrong – good from bad – or even cares. It just takes what you tell it to do and reacts.

The more you tell it to repeat the same function, the more it reacts the same way. This eventually forms a thick, long-term memory pattern called a habit.

We must form habits in order to live. Imagine getting up tomorrow and not remembering how to brush your teeth, shower, dress, tie your shoes, eat with a fork or spoon, operate the car or computer, tell time, or use the phone.

By the time you re-taught yourself, the day would be over and the process would start all over again. Habits thus mold our everyday world, and since we need habits to survive, once you form a habit, the subconscious mind will do all in its power to hold that habit, whether good or bad. Why?

"The subconscious just reacts to what it is told." Since the subconscious mind is older and, as you have read, the seniority system works with brain function, the subconscious will always overrule the conscious mind. Your *willpower* will eventually lose to a far older function. This tug-of-war thus continues unless you gain the

knowledge to bring the conscious and subconscious mind together in unison.

Imagination

In the late 1700s, the physician Charles d'Elson remarked: "If the medicine of imagination is best, why should we not practice the medication of imagination?"

Two great leaders have known the power of imagination. The French general *Napoleon* understood the benefits of focusing the mind when he wrote in his memoirs, "Imagination rules the world." In the early 1900s, Albert Einstein remarked, "Imagination is more powerful than knowledge."

These two men of vision – one attempting to conquer the world with an army of obedience, the other to conquer the universe using pencil and equations – both knew the challenge that lay in observing victory within the mind's imagination. Knowledge falls on deaf ears without imagination to grasp and understand.

Imagination, the ability to foresee our future destiny from the moment we become self-aware, rules our existence. The dreams of what we might achieve, our successes, failures, even what lies beyond death, sets humans apart.

This destiny, however, may become clouded and changed by untimely sensitive emotional events that can form negative habits.

We are exposed to many perils in life, both physical and psychological. We have the knowledge to impart, and we know why and how reactions occur, but transferring that knowledge without imagination can form negative habits that can be silent killers. These habits dwell in the subconscious, and slowly and methodically control the mind both chemically and emotionally. They are not evil, but just react to fulfill an obligation you unknowingly created. One might perceive a negative habit as: *"Something I just can't break." "I'm addicted to it." "You have to die of something."* or *"I just don't care."*

Note: Imagination is therefore an important tool in controlling your fat storage. Using your imagination positively can change your body structure, health, and even your outlook on life.

R.L. Erickson C.H.P.

SECTION THREE

Medications and The Body's Energy Saving Controls

R.L. Erickson C.H.P.

8

Medications or Legal Poisons?

R.L. Erickson C.H.P.

Evolution of Medications

Have you ever asked yourself how our ancestors survived for multi-millennia of years with all sorts of ailments and, unlike what we have been led to believe, lived long and healthy lives, when a staggering ninety percent of the medications on the markets today have been invented within the last 75 years?

Compounding (making prescription medications) was believed to have been started in antiquity by shamans, medicine men, and later the clergy. These compounds were usually naturally occurring herbs, plants, alcohol, sulfur, and/or opiates, along with chants to remove the demons and bad spirits from the body.

Evidence dating back 5,000 years have the Greeks and Egyptians developing Sleep Temples – a combination of herb therapy and what we refer to today as hypnosis was employed to allow the body's own healing mechanism (our auto-immune system) time to repair itself.

Specialization of compounding, around the ninth century, in and around Baghdad (Iraq), quickly spread to Europe in the form of alchemy (the beginnings of modern chemistry), which slowly evolved as early physicians began to abandon beliefs of demonic possession for a more scientific approach, leading to a new industry: that of pharmacy.

The pharmacy profession, as populations grew and physicians had less time to prepare medications for their patient, soon began to compound medicines for many doctors. This separation of duties continued to grow until the 1800s, when the pharmacist was acknowledged as a compounder of medications and the physician as the therapist.

In the 1950s, commercial pharmaceutical manufacturers began producing medications in mass doses and the pharmacy profession was reduced to dispensing medications, and became a liaison between the drug makers and the physician.

The 1990s saw the Food and Drug Administration (FDA) put certain drugs on a fast track for approval as fierce competition between manufacturers and the public's needs grew. This has led to the unethical release of many medications before adequate research has been preformed.

There are countless examples, as evidenced by certain prescription drugs prematurely released and later proven deadly, including drugs for: dieting (fen-phen, Redux), antibiotics (Raxar), blood pressure (Posicor), pain (Duract), diabetes (Rezulin), cholesterol (baycol), and nighttime heartburn (Propulsid). Many chemical formulas that were touted as "miracle drugs" have, over –time, proved to be fatal poisons, the consequences of which we still are feeling today.

Note: *the term "Alternative Medicine" has, until recently, reflected a negative connotation in the medical community. To this author taking a man-made pill is the alternative, especially if it can result in serious side effects or death.*

Obesity Medications

Development of obesity medications has led many to believe in a "Magic fat loss Pill". To date, no such pill exists, and the side effects to many of these drugs are very dangerous, as demonstrated by fen – phen and Redux-related deaths and the subsequent removal of these and other drugs from the market.

Most obesity drugs mimic or attempt to enhance chemicals found naturally in our brain, especially in the hypothalamus. The main function of the hypothalamus is *Homeostasis,* or maintaining the body's status quo. The hypothalamus has the ability to control and holds to a precise value the body's endocrine system, blood pressure, body temperature, metabolism, adrenaline levels, fluids, electrolyte balance, and body weight. Collectively these are called the set points.

Although these set points can increase or decrease over time, from day to day they are remarkably fixed. The more dangerous obesity drugs attempt to alter the set point for weight and fat storage, attempting to lower the weight of an individual.

The problem, however, is two-fold. These drugs often have adverse side effects that may alter a different set point that the Hypothalamus controls. This function may be unrelated to weigh but essential for survival. Second, these drugs may alter or induce muscle loss, creating a long-term decrease in the muscle–to-fat ratio as weight loss occurs.

Scientist within the pharmaceutical industry have concentrated on five strategies for primary drug action that might lead to significant weight loss:

1. Appetite suppressants

2. Inhibitors of fat absorption

3. Increased thermogenesis (releasing food energy as heat without requiring increases in physical activity)

4. Stimulators of fat or protein metabolism

5. Modulators regulating body weight

Most marketed obesity drugs are appetite suppressants that act directly on the central nervous system (CNS) and reduce food intake by modulating the concentrations of the neurotransmitters (Serotonin and Noradrenaline) in the brain. Many so-called thermogenic over-the-counter supplements have little or no long-term value.

What does all this technical jargon mean? We are being trained to become dependent on a pill that attempts to regulate that which has taken multi-millennia of evolution to perfect: our natural internal bodily functions.

A pill may one day solve all our problems of appetite, emotions, and habits, but why wait? These functions will usually perform normally if you lower internal stress and control daily Calories intake.

The Tainted Scientific Method

With the advent of science and its precise calculations, man quickly recognized that personal and cultural beliefs influence both our perceptions and our interpretations of natural phenomena; scientists thus adopted a step-by-step procedure call the scientific method.

The scientific method is a process by which scientists, collectively and over time; endeavor to construct an accurate, consistent and non-arbitrary representation of the world. The scientific method attempts, therefore, to minimize the influence of bias or prejudice in the experimenter when testing a hypothesis or a theory. This is accomplished in a four-step process.

The four basic steps:

1. Observe and describe an event or group of events.

2. Formulate a hypothesis (idea) to explain the event.

3. Test your hypothesis to see if it explains the event or if it creates new event(s).

4. Have several independent experimenters perform your hypothesis to see if they obtain the same results.

If the experiments bear out the hypothesis it may come to be regarded as a theory or law of nature. If the experiments do not bear out the hypothesis, *it must be rejected or modified.*

A major problem with the scientific method has arisen over the last 30 years, as many unsubstantiated hypothesis *have not been rejected or modified.*

First: The primary reason for this misinformation is that experiments are done by authority figures that try to establish a *hypothetical belief as truth.* Thus, any hypothesis that has been observed by so-called *independent research* suddenly becomes a proven theory or truth.

Second: The most fundamental error is to mistake the hypothesis for an explanation of an event, without performing experimental tests. Sometimes common sense and logic tempt us into believing that testing is simply *not needed.*

There are always possibilities that new observations or new experiments will conflict with long-standing theory, however, every day, hundreds of companies use commercials to sell various products using this misinformation technique. The very fundamental primus of the scientific method has been distorted.

Third: Errors in miscommunication and competition force scientists to rely only on their company data. Scientists may feel internal or external pressures to get a specific result in a timely manner, or have strong beliefs that their hypothesis is true.

Competition among companies working on the same product shuts off communication between scientists, because billions of dollars may ride on a specific drug, medical procedure, or device.

These companies may ignore or rule out data that does not support their therapy hypothesis in order to get a product to market; negative results, which were missed by experimenters whose data contained flaws, are simply explained away as a systematic background error.

The scientific method has been tainted in this modern age. The very fact that a drug has to be prescribed should alert the public. Buyers beware.

9

The Body's Energy Saving Controls

R.L. Erickson C.H.P.

"Laws of Nature"

Our prehistoric ancestors evolved consuming foods that occurred naturally, which were higher in fiber (ungrounded grains, tubers, grasses, and nuts), lower in fat (wild animals have much lower fat than our domesticated breeding stock), and without chemical enhancements or genetic engineering.

In our current environment of engineered foods and social problems, our digestive system, stress, and habits have altered our nutritional and weight set points. No longer do we store the majority of excess fat for starvation episodes, as our ancestors did. Today's fast paced emotional stress- and money-oriented society has the majority of excess fat being stored for perceived or imagined protection rather than for actual events.

This change still works within the framework of our genetics. Genetics still plays a major role in how we store fat. Therefore, not every person can be at his or her medical ideal weight. Each individual should thus set a desired comfort weight goal.

Understanding the laws of nature, especially the law of conservation thermodynamics, which state that *the amount of energy in the universe is always the same, and can neither be increased nor lessened,* applies to all things in the universe including our calorie intake. Since nature usually takes the path of least resistance, if we do not use the energy we consume, we will either excrete as waste or store as body fat what is left over, whichever takes less energy.

It is often easier to excrete excess protein as ureic acid than to convert it to fat. It is usually easier to convert energy foods – carbohydrates and fats – to stored body fat than to excrete it in our feces. These laws give insight as to how our body treats food, and makes it easy to understand that it is not what, when, or how you eat, but the quantity of foods in proper daily amounts.

Weight Is Not The Problem?

For many years, healthcare professionals have tried to teach the public that the *key* to losing weight is consuming fewer calories. This "calories in, calories out" philosophy loses meaning when we know that the *key* is to understand that **Fat** is the problem, not **Weight**.

Weight charts used by physicians and insurance companies are based on mortality graphs. Mortality graphs help actuaries (people that compile insurance statistics) to calculate, using the Law of Large Numbers theory, a profitable price for life insurance policies.

Mortality graphs show statistical death rates of individuals in a number of categories: male, female, origins, smoker, medical condition, occupation, heredity, and weight, to name a few. These graphs are good indicators because they are based on a large population number kept over many years.

Note: What is ideal for the pricing of life insurance may not be ideal for your weight.

When you go to the doctor for an examination, usually you are weighed and then given your BMI (Body Mass Index) number. This number is derived as follows: BMI = 704 x Weight/ divided by (Height x Height), where weight is in pounds and height is in inches.

A reading of 24-26 is considered marginally overweight, 26-29.9 overweight, and readings of 30 or more are considered obese. *BMI is not, in my opinion, a good indicator for obesity, because BMI measures your entire body weight. It does not take into account muscle, bone, or necessary liquid weight.*

Health problems arise when individuals store excess body fat. Type 2 diabetes, high blood pressure, cancer, heart disease, arthritis, sleep apnea, and asthma start with higher than normal triglycerides and blood sugars. Excess body fat, not weight, thus encourages these civilized diseases.

Weight alone is misleading. Mortality and BMI charts lump everyone into one classification, regardless of muscle structure. Would you say Arnold Schwarzenegger was obese?

Body fat tests are more indicative in determining obesity. They require extra effort by a medical practitioner that simply hasn't the time or equipment to perform body fat tests. Body fat in excess of 31% for a female and 26% for a male would be considered obese regardless of her/his weight-to-height ratio.

In attempting to reach what your physician describes as your "ideal weight" in these mortality charts, many people resort to taking thermogenic prescribed medications and/or starting a crash weight-loss diet.

Every day, somewhere in America, this play is repeated over and over again. *Does this play sound familiar?*

Act 10, take 6: the Crash Diet – The Ultimate Yo-yo Plan!!

<u>Scene set-up</u>: You are in your bedroom, readying for work. It is the sixth day of fad diet #10, the Ultimate Yo-yo Plan...aaaaand <u>ACTION!</u> -*That little voice in your brain (literally because of our hypothalamus) has been chemically telling you to eat, but you have willpower this time and it is strong, so you resist temptation.*

<u>Time lapse:</u> The weeks go by, and all of a sudden you are starting to see results. One pound, three pounds, eight pounds, twenty pounds – wow, you are ecstatic. *"This undoubtedly is the most wonderful,*

best diet in the world. I want to go on TV and do a testimonial for this new fantastic YO-YO Plan." "Yes, it was worth all the pain I endured! I'm losing weight!" "But, wait! What weight – fat, water, or muscle?" "Oh, well, I don't care. I am losing the weight."

Again, a time lapse as we jump forward eight months.

Act 11, take 7: the Crash Diet – Reaction

Scene set-up: Talking to your friend eight months later. ACTION: *"Yes, Mary that diet was great! I just wish I had stuck with it; then, I might not have gained all that weight plus three pounds back again."*

Fad crash diets don't work. Yes, you had willpower: you didn't eat for all those weeks and you lost weight. The only problem: you weren't eating, but your body was. It literally was eating you, only it wasn't eating fat as you had hoped; it was eating non-essential calorie-burning muscle. So, in the end you gained all the weight back in the form excess body fat, lowering your *muscle-to-fat ratio*, and thus your metabolism.

Another very popular crash weight loss diet on the market today has a physician controlling a very low fat, low calorie program. You are given a standard exam including blood work, weighed once a week while listening to pep talks from a personal trainer or nurse, and sold prepackaged food. You will lose weight – usually from your wallet – between $3,700 and $6,500 worth of weight, in fact!

Other well-known crash weight loss diets also offer prepackaged foods at tremendous mark-ups. Some crash weight loss diets don't even let you eat real food. They sell you on often horrible tasting liquid refreshments, which are usually a diuretic and/or laxative.

It is little wonder that 70+% of dieters gain back more weight than they lost after they quit a diet program.

Set Points: The Starvation Response Mode

An understanding of homeostasis (remaining constant), set points, and the body's starvation response mechanism and how to control their effects is helpful to this or any nutritional program. In general, the reason most diets fail is the body's ancestral starvation response mechanism and the conservation gene.

Homeostasis is a corrective mechanism that uses a process called *negative feedback* to ensure conditions remain favorable for health. The hypothalamus acts as a conductor, fine-tuning the body with "receptors" and "effectors" that bring about a reaction. We call these reactive points *–set points*.

Set points attempt to maintain the status quo, so that the body can work at top efficiency levels. However, it can only work within tolerable limits. Under extreme conditions, like continuous overeating, set points can be disabled by channeling signals through the *autonomic nervous system* and hormone messengers. The negative feedback mechanism is shut down, and set points are then changed to reflect the new environment.

If a person continues to consume excess calories, their maximum weight set point will increase. Each new maximum becomes a new set point. This can have an adverse effect on bodily function.

When a person starts a low calorie crash diet, the body first reacts to the sudden decrease in energy input by causing the pancreas to secrete an enzyme alerting the liver to release glucose into the body to try to keep the set point energy levels constant.

As time passes and we continue a very low calorie diet, the hypothalamus activates the pituitary gland of our endocrine system to encourage a change in our hunger patterns, emotions, sleep, and metabolism. This can lead to a lower overall set point in metabolism, which in some cases is irrevocable. Moods, emotions, brain function, sleep, and stress also are affected.

Very low calorie, prolonged fad diets can result in serious side effects and even death. Often before this happens, the hypothalamus calls upon an ancient and little know conservation gene to save the day.

The Conservation Gene

If all tactics by the hypothalamus's starvation response fail to stimulate increased food consumption because, "you have willpower", our little friend the *conservation gene* steps forward. Genes are in every cell of the body so you are up against over 4 trillion competitors for energy. Recent studies are confirming the fact we indeed have an ancient friend called a conservation gene. This gene is thought to be a throwback to our prehistoric days, when we could only forage within a small geographical area. It helped conserve consumed energy in times of famine or hardship, such as extended illness, accidents, and harsh climatic changes, where feeding might be impossible, scarce, or completely unavailable for an extended time. Some scientists have even hypothesized that this gene could have evolved from an even more ancient hibernation state.

With the vast quantities of food at our disposal today this gene has little to do, but it can have devastating consequences for a quick-fix crash dieter.

The conservation gene has one main function —conserve energy. When all set point systems fail to conserve energy during a *real or perceived* starvation event, the following orders are released by the conservation gene, and strictly obeyed:

1. Slow down all non-essential mechanisms

2. Convert all excess muscle tissue to energy

3. Excrete all excess water weight

4. Lower all brain function

5. Increase hunger drive

6. Lower emotional energy output

7. Conserve all body fat energy reserves for future use

Note: When a dieter awakens the conservation gene they have lost the "war of willpower". The conservation gene is way older and has too much control for you to win; it simply informs the body to start consuming itself.

Keeping The Conservation Gene Dormant

Understanding the starvation response mode, the hypothalamus set points, and the conservation gene allows one to accomplished the task of weight loss rather easily.

First: The hypothalamus is very stingy about its set points, so it takes some repeated coaxing to change them. In the event of perceived starvation due to lower caloric intake, the hypothalamic response has a delay switch of four to five days, another evolutionary wonder. This delaying mechanism evolved to make allowances for the effects of sickness, injury, or sudden climatic changes (e.g. flooding) on our prehistoric ancestors, when hunting food may have been impossible for a few days.

For example, if you were consuming an average of 3400 calories per day and started a 1200-calorie per day crash weight diet, your body would offer no hypothalamus response for the first three to five days (the delay window).

If, however, you continued on this 1200-calorie per day diet, the hypothalamus would assume food was becoming scarce and the starvation response mode would be activated. After the starvation response mechanism was activated and you still failed to respond (i.e. increase your calorie intake) to the signals set into motion, the hypothalamus would then activate the conservation gene and it would issue its strict orders.

Second: Using this delaying mechanism to our advantage, we can step the amounts of calories and nutrients each day over a seven-day period. In a sense, chemically tricking the brain. Then, by simply repeating the process over and over each week, the hypothalamus will not "switch on" the starvation response mode or induce the conservation gene.

As long as you keep the starvation response mechanism in the "off" position the conservation gene will never be activated. Remember, the conservation gene is only activated by the hypothalamus, and only after the starvation response mechanism has failed. *You will thus be able to continue to cannibalize body fat for energy and conserve muscle tissue.* By repeating this process over and over each week, the body will naturally, easily, and safely consume the body fat it has stored for what it perceives to be just such an occasion. You lose "dangerous" levels of stored body fat, while feeling great. Your body and mind are rewarded, and all because you have learned this little secret.

You may continue to eat all the foods you enjoy, anytime you want, prepared however you want, and at the same time convert stored body fat into the energy needed to run your body at its maximum.

So What Took So Long?

For years, the medical community, the government, national health organizations, educators, employers, family, friends, spouses, and even our children have bombarded us with misinformation concerning food. They are not being mean, but merely repeating half-truths and misinformation that they were taught again and again. I am reminded of a famous Western movie in which a newspaperman says: "When the legend become the truth, print the legend." Unfortunately the legend concerning food, steeped in half-truths over the last 30 years, has become the truth.

In the introduction to this book, I stated that I am not your doctor. My concern, however, is to offer you a nutritional program that will allow you to lose stored body fat easily and effectively, while increasing the muscle-to-fat ratio, restoring your body's natural metabolic rate for continued good health.

This program is not a diet in the traditional sense. Diets are quick fixes to a life-long problem. The New Millennium Diet is a part of a larger program. It allows you to fit your lifestyle into a nutritional program that you can live with for your entire life. Imagine living healthily five, ten, or even twenty years longer than you would have had you not started this program. A happier, more energetic and enjoyable future awaits you, with a stronger sense of self-esteem and self-worth.

You are probably asking yourself; why haven't there been hundreds of books written on the subject? Why is this not the standard health guide? These are all valid questions – I asked them myself.

The simple answer is MONEY!

This program has you buying:

- <u>NO</u> prescription medication, medical device, or procedure

- <u>NO</u> exercise machines

- <u>NO</u> package of videotapes

- <u>NO</u> Prepackaged special foods

- <u>NO</u> one-on-one phone bank

- <u>NO</u> daily supplement powder, bar, or tablet

The monetary food chain previously discussed is not satisfied with merely receiving royalties from one book and audio CD when billions can be made from expensive or repeat sales.

SECTION FOUR

The New Millennium Diet Step by Step

R.L. Erickson C.H.P.

10

Reversing Habitual Eating Syndrome

R.L. Erickson C.H.P.

A Quick Glance

This program is designed to reverse our altered our fat storage mechanism of excess body fat as protection against socioeconomic stress. *The New Millennium Diet* gives the reader the following:

First: internal stress reduction can be achieved though daily relaxation methods. The authors guided imagery relaxation weight loss <u>CD</u> is strongly recommended, as it is designed especially for those with *Habitual Eating Syndrome*. Other methods include meditation or exercise. As stress is reduced, so, too, will your need for excess calorie consumption.

Second: Use of the pre-calculated *Seven-Day revolving Step Rate Calorie program,* allows you to lose excess body fat without burning muscle. Increasing your, daily calorie intake over a seven-day period then repeating the process steps-up fat burning, while keeping the starvation response mode and conservation gene dormant. This process reverses the muscle to fat ratio raising the basal metabolic rate (BMR). You start losing weight *immediately* as more fat is used for energy, even while you are sleeping.

To determine your pre-calculated revolving daily step rate calorie maximums simply follow the pre-calculated charts by:

1. Choosing your own comfort weight.

2. Determine your base number.

3. Determine you activity level inactive, average, active

Once you have your *Seven-Day Step Rate Calorie Maximums,* use the *New Multiple Calorie Chart*, and *Sample Menus* provided to help you stay within your daily calorie range. Enjoy mixing and matching

117

new foods, as you eat four to seven meals per day. By continuing to use the relaxation weight loss audio CD and follow the Seven-Day revolving Step Rate Calorie program weekly, you can expect the following results:

- Correct weight loss

- Decrease in stress levels, feeling fuller with less food

- New lower weight set point

- Muscle-to-fat ratio increase

- Basal Metabolic rate increase

- Improved energy levels

- Optimal brain functioning

- Better sleep patterns

- Alleviation of stomach and intestinal discomfort

- Enhanced and fortified emotions and immune system

- Decrease in colds, flu, back pain and headaches

- Increased self-esteem and self-worth

The following steps will give you a more in-depth look into *The New Millennium Diet and reversing Habitual Eating Syndrome.*

Counteracting Negative Stress, Emotions and Habits

We face challenges every day that our ancestors never dreamed possible: frivolous lawsuits, bigotry and hatred, terrorism. Add to that the stress of automobiles, planes, mass transit, line management issues, monetary concerns, politics, marriage, single parenting, hospital stays, prescription medicine reactions, drug use, crime, smoking, alcoholism, social diseases, obesity, plus instant around the world news of violence, catastrophe, war, and senseless victimization.

These and other socioeconomic stressors have caused us to gain weight for protection against perceived, imaginary, and/or real threats, as the very foundations we hold as truths and mainstays to morality that surround our everyday lives are changing.

In order to lessen the effects of these stressors, many individuals have turned to prescription medicines. Unfortunately, the side effects can be as bad or worse than the stress. Some anxiety and depression medications actually enhance body fat production.

Three processes—guided imagery, meditation, and exercise can produce natural stress relieving chemicals to counteract the imbalance stress hormones often create. These relaxation effectors can be released in times of stress to help nullify the stress hormone reactions.

The benefits of exercise are well known and when combined with either guided imagery or meditation can be very effective. If however, exercise does not fit your lifestyle. You may want to explore meditation and guided imagery separately, as these two methods can be very effective and preformed while sitting or lying down.

Meditation occurs in the conscious mind and therefore is somewhat less effective as true relaxation. In meditation, one uses a thought or word to concentrate thinking about change or just relaxing. The stress is thus lowered but, as long as you are in your conscious mind, the short-term working memory remains "switched on" and continues to create "noise", often blocking the relaxation. The following is an effective meditation device to lower stress.

Meditation Stress Reduction Passage

Place yourself in a comfortable position. You may listen to low soft back-round music or just silence. Close you eyes and concentrate on and a setting that make you feel relaxed: beach—pond—mountain stream—back yard—woods or garden park.

Now starting at your feet, tense each part of your body, for a count of five, then slowly relax it: Feet—legs—buttocks—stomach—back—chest—shoulders—arms—hands—neck—face. As you tense and relax, tense and relax, imagine the place in your mind becoming more vivid to you. Leave your chair and travel into this setting in your mind, and as you do feel all the stress leaving your muscle moving out through the skin, and out into space, like little golden sparkles—away—away—away.

Learning Guided imagery using autosuggestion from a person or CD is a far superior counterbalance to stress-related conditions. Guided imagery fits within the science of hypnosis. Hypnosis has for years been considered the "bad boy" of psychotherapy, primarily because of three events which started in the mid1800s:

1. The very name 'hypnosis' coined in 1850 by Dr. James Braid, after the Greek god of sleep Ypnos. The name represents the look of a person in hypnosis (as if asleep or in a trance) rather than explaining the science.

2. Sigmund Freud often referred to, as the father of modern psychology, who studied under Charcot (a famous hypnotist), was a bad hypnotist. He subsequently abandoned it for his psychoanalysis principles. In his later years Freud did finally endorsed hypnosis, but the damage to the science had already occurred.

3. Most people associate hypnosis with the antics of stage, movie, and cults that use hypnosis to seemingly make people do things against their will.

It wasn't until World War II and the Korean conflict, when the military ran low on morphine, that hypnosis revived its potential through its use on the battlefield for pain control and shell shock.

Today increased popularity of alternatives to medication has continued to raise awareness of this science. Today, we regard hypnosis as: *a naturally occurring phenomenon that counteracts stress by any form that alters consciousness through attention (focusing the mind), to the subconscious; thus allowing change through our imagination.*

Hypnosis has a higher efficacy than that of meditation because it works in the subconscious (limbic system), where emotions, habits, and perceptions are formed. In the hypnotic state, focusing the mind becomes more pronounced because one bypasses the conscious state and thus the "noise of consciousness" (short-term memory), and works in the older sub-conscious area of the mind.

This state is sometimes referred to as a focused attention state, allowing one to focus on specific ideas or events. The calming effect is caused by the release of the effectors dopamine and endorphins as the body prepares for what it perceives as readying for sleep. These powerful agents, sometimes referred to as the "opiates of the body", nullify the stress effectors adrenaline and cortisol.

While in this focused attention phase, one can effectively, accomplish through imagination, changes in his or her outlook on life by correcting negative stored emotions and habits.

Learning a form of autosuggestion (self-hypnosis) from a, qualified hypnotist practitioner enhances efficacy. Since all hypnotic techniques are ultimately autosuggestion (made by the individual), the hypnotist mainly instructs the patient on how to achieve the hypnotic state rather than having the patient read a book on the subject. The hypnotist teaches autosuggestion techniques so the patient can learn how to return to this state on their own. As the hypnotic state is repeated, it becomes easier and affords more positive results often completely changing a person's perceived or real negative outlook and promoting a healthy lifestyle.

I have created an audio relaxation weight loss CD. This audio CD will help you learn how to relax effectively, thus nullifying stress. You can use this CD in the comfort of your own home, at work, or in any safe relaxing area.

You may wish to listen to the CD individually, with a family member, or in a small support group. As stress levels, perceptions, negative habits, and emotions are controlled, the need to continue to use fat as protection diminishes and over eating urges decrease.

Determine Your Comfort Weight

Your weight should be a weight that makes you feel comfortable. I trust the earlier statement concerning excess body fat verses weight was noted; however, I understand weight is still the main issue, and can involve a series of learned psychological issues dictated again by social interactions.

- Some women, for example, want to weigh under a set poundage amount because they believe going over that amount means they are fat.

- Some short people use weight as a way to compensate for height. Weight takes up space. Size is power.

- Some equate health to weight. A chunky baby is a healthy baby.

- Some imagine overweight people as jollier (Jolly Old Saint Nick).

- Some believe being overweight equates to personal wealth.

These perceptions only increase the problems. *Reality check*: Excess stored body fat can lead to pain, ill health, and premature death.

Note: Do you know of any obese person that ever celebrated their 100th birthday?

The nutritionist's standard for normal stored body fat is one month. This equates to a body fat percentage amount for women of 19-24% and for men of 14-19% these amounts will rise with age if muscle atrophies from lower physical activity.

Mortality tables are merely starting points. Your comfort weight may be several pounds higher that what is shown on these charts. Remember mortality charts are for determining insurance premiums not your weight. You are ultimately in control. Determine a weight that makes you feel good, have the ability to see as a future attainable goal, and then let achieving that goal be your main objective.

Establish Your Base Number *and* The Daily Calorie Profile

When the amount of calories consumed is equal to or greater than the body's daily needs, we remain in status quo or store the excess calories as fat. In order to lose excess body fat, we need to eat the right amount of food each day to adequately supply our body with nutrients, and at the same time eat less calories than our body needs to maintain our current status quo, so that the difference in calories can be used from our fat stores. This takes some fine-tuning to keep the starvation response mechanism switched off. The calculation charts provided help to determine your specific *base number*.

The base number has been extrapolated to reflect an average calorie requirement per day for a total body weight over a seven-day period. It was designed to then step rate this average over this seven-day period. By adjusting, to reflect the activity level of the particular individual, we keep the starvation response mechanism switched off.

Factors contributing to calorie daily assignments include:

- Time frame for your fat loss (3-6-12 mo.)

- Age-adjusted Basal Metabolic Rate (BMR)

- Gender (male or female)

- Physical activity (inactive, average, active)

- Weight (fat-to-muscle ratio)

Time frame: It takes time to lose body fat, and my calculations are based on a 12-month formula. Realizing, however, that most people want results in a shorter time frame, I have adjusted the calorie intake accordingly, with emphasis again on keeping the starvation response mechanism switched off. The shorter formulas of 3 and 6 months are especially beneficial if 10-50 pounds is the amount of loss desired.

Age is a factor in BMR. Studies have confirmed that our metabolism slows starting around age 27 and slowly drops until it tends to level off in our late 60s. Consideration of this phenomenon (mainly caused by muscle atrophy from non-exercise) has been incorporated into my calculations. BMR charts are also misleading because they use the total body weight in their calculations. It must be noted that one cannot eat the calories assessed by a BMR chart and lose weight. Adjustments have been made in this area.

Gender: Men, on average, have more muscle tissue than women. Muscle is the main calorie burning tissue in our body; therefore men burn more calories than women. My calculations have allowed for this gender difference in the weight columns by increasing the weight differentials for each base number.

Physical activity: The more you involve the muscle in everyday activity, the more calories you burn. Low impact resistance training is especially desirable in replacing fat with muscle and avoiding strain and injury to the joints.

On the base number charts, I have allowed for activity by offering three categories: the *inactive* or sedentary person (little or no extra activity), the *average* person, (yard or garden work and/or exercising three times per week), and the *active* person (an exercise routine consisting, in addition to your normal activities, of at least four sessions per week for a minimum duration of 50 minutes per session).

Note: The body adjusts over time to work performed. It is important to realize that, even though housework, childcare, and your job may be very strenuous, your body adapts to this work, making exercise most important. If, however, you refuse to exercise, you will still lose weight if you choose the <u>inactive</u> maximum daily calorie amounts.

125

Weight: The more muscle you have on your body, the more calories you burn. Muscle burns about 1.28 calories per kilogram, which translates to about 15 calories per pound per day. As we age our activity levels usually drop, and muscles atrophy (get smaller), while fat is stored in ever increasing amounts as protection against stress. This multiplier effect, as stated earlier, leads to a *drop in the muscle-to-fat ratio*. Since fat is excess stored energy, very few calories are needed to retain it on our body. This can lead to consuming literally thousands of extra, unneeded calories per day. Base number adjustments have been made in the weight categories to compensate for lower than average lean muscle-to-fat ratios.

Finding your base number: All the calculations have been completed for you to find your *base number* on the following corresponding charts. You need only select the time frame for weight loss, and then locate your base number by your gender, age, and weight.

For example:

Time frame**:** six months

Gender: female

Age: 38

Weight: 224

Go to the Six Month Plan chart for women; look for your age and weight group (age group = 27-42 weight group = 201-285). Your base number is: **7**

Finding your daily calorie maximums: Proceed with your base number to the revolving *Daily Calorie Maximum* charts to determine your *daily calorie maximums.*

For example, if your base number is **7 and you** weigh 224, your revolving daily calorie maximums are as follows:

Base 7
Wt. 218-247

	Day 1	Day 2	Day 3	Day 4	Day 5	Day 6	Day 7
Inactive	1100	1440	1615	1885	1910	1960	2130
Average	1200	1540	1715	1985	2010	2060	2230
Active	1400	1740	1885	2085	2210	2260	2430

As you will note, calculations for activity levels have been made in the *inactive, average,* and *active* categories. (Remember the criteria for your status.)

By repeating the process every seven days we chemically trick the body keeping it out of the starvation response zone. Stored Body fat is now consumed instead of muscle.

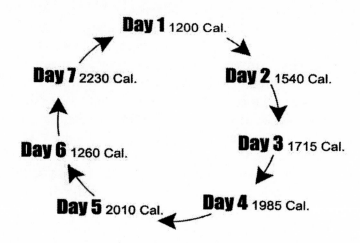

Eat all the calories up to this maximum of your daily calorie intake. It is important not to exceed your daily calorie maximum by more than 150 calories per day, and eating 300 calories below your maximum each day could switch on the starvation response mechanism.

- *NOTE: If you are within 200 calories of your total weekly calorie maximum and you did not lose weight, drop back one space on your base number. Example; (**Base number 7** –average— drops back to **Base number 7** –inactive— on your daily calorie maximums).*

Establish Your Daily Meals

The food industry spends millions of dollars each year to develop bio-engineered foods that have the right texture, smell, and taste These foods, eaten in large portions, show up in the form of excess body fat. In determining your daily meal programs remember, food is only a transport mechanism of energy and nutrients, concentrating on proper calorie daily intake is the first step in controlling you weight.

Staying within your revolving daily calorie maximums allows you to eat the foods you enjoy while losing weight. This sometimes may seem to be a problem when considering that many fast foods contain over 1000 calories per serving. You may still eat these types of foods. Just stay within your daily calorie maximum, and consume them over the day instead of eating them in one sitting. You can also satisfy your cravings for taste, texture, and smell by substituting similar food items. As an example, one Hardee's *Monster Burger* weighs 288 grams and contains 1060 calories. A Hardee's *Famous Star* weighs 245 grams and has 570 calories. And two regular Hardee's hamburgers are 540 calories at 220 grams. You get the taste, texture, and smell of Hardee's, and approximately the same amount of food by weight but at half the calories.

Eating small meals throughout the day is also helpful when considering that you expend 8-10 % of your daily energy output to digest the foods you eat. If you are constantly digesting food, you are constantly burning excess calories.

You are now ready to get started with your calorie chart, but the problem with most typical calorie charts is the way they list foods and calories. Most merely copy the United States Department of Agriculture's charts, which show the food type, portion size, calories, and fat per serving. They really don't look at reality situations.

This can be very frustrating if, for example, while dining out and you forgot your calculator. The calorie charts contained in this book have foods divided not only by groups but also by calorie per meal size. For example, an 8 oz. Porterhouse steak consists of 680 calories, or one *Egg McMuffin* is 300 calories. You may also compare foods with similar calories in the same calorie range. Suppose you want to try some different foods but are reluctant because you are not familiar with their calorie amount. These charts will easily allow you to compare different foods. For example, *Pizza Hut* Thin'n' Crispy w/Chicken Supreme (medium pizza) 1 slice 113 grams. A *Subway* 6" Veggie Delite Sub 163 grams, and *Wendy's* Hidden Valley Ranch Dressing (1pkt) 57 grams, all contain two hundred Calories.

These charts are simplistic and more in tune with your eating profile.

Although there are thousands of different foods to choose from, most people settle for about 17 favorites. These staples of your everyday consumption are a great starting point in determining your daily calorie meal structure.

This text provides you with a favorite food profile sheet. Simply list your favorite foods plus any foods you would be interested in incorporating into your meal profile. Once you have determined the types of foods you want and enjoy, you can easily and simply determine your daily meals.

It will not take much time to start memorizing calories of the foods you enjoy. By mapping out the foods you enjoy, you will be more likely to stay on track.

Note: *It will soon become second nature to look at food from its calorie amount rather than taste and texture, because you are not limiting yourself to the types of foods you can eat. No longer do you need to worry about the fat content, protein, or carbohydrates. Eat the foods you enjoy, experiment with different foods, and enjoy eating as you always did but now, by staying within your daily calorie maximum, body fat weight loss will occur.*

SECTION FIVE

Charts Comfort Weight, Base Numbers, Daily Calorie Maximums, Calories and Sample Menus

R.L. Erickson C.H.P.

WEIGHT TABLES

R.L. Erickson C.H.P.

The following weight charts are actually insurance mortality tables for comparison only. Your comfort weight may be several pounds higher.

Ideal (?) Height & Weight Table

WOMEN

(Clothing weighing 3 lbs. in shoes with 1" heels)

Height in feet and inches	Weight in pounds
4' 10"	102-131
4' 11"	103-134
5' 0"	104-137
5' 1"	106-140
5' 2"	108-143
5' 3"	111-147
5' 4"	114-151
5' 5"	117-155
5' 6"	120-159
5' 7"	123-163
5' 8"	126-167
5' 9"	129-170
5' 10"	132-173
5' 11"	135-176
6' 0"	138-179

MEN

(Clothing weighing 5 lbs. in shoes with 1" heels)

Height in feet and inches	Weight in pounds
5' 2"	128-150
5' 3"	130-153
5' 4"	132-156
5' 5"	134-160
5' 6"	136-164
5' 7"	138-168
5' 8"	140-172
5' 9"	142-176
5' 10"	144-180
5' 11"	146-184
6' 0"	149-188
6' 1"	152-192
6' 2"	155-197
6' 3"	158-202
6' 4"	162-207

BASE NUMBERS

WOMEN AND MEN

R.L. Erickson C.H.P.

Finding Your Base Number

The following charts are designed by the duration of your weight loss program. Be realistic in your time frame.

WOMEN

3-MONTH WEIGHT LOSS PLAN – base number

	Under 185	186-200	201-285	286+
Age 10-26	9	8	7	6
Age 27-42	8	7	6	5
Age 43+	8	7	5	5

WOMEN

6-MONTH WEIGHT LOSS PLAN – base number

	Under 185	186-200	201-285	286+
Age 10-26	10	9	8	7
Age 27-42	9	8	7	6
Age 43+	8	7	6	5

WOMEN

1+ YEAR WEIGHT LOSS PLAN – base number

	Under 185	186-200	201-285	286-312	380+
Age 10-26	11	10	9	8	7
Age 27-42	10	9	8	7	6
Age 43+	9	8	7	6	5

MEN

The following charts are designed by the duration of your weight loss program. Be realistic in your time frame.

3-MONTH WEIGHT LOSS PLAN – base number

	Under 205	206-280	281-320	321+
Age 10-26	9	8	7	6
Age 27-42	8	7	6	5
Age 43+	7	6	5	5

MEN

6-MONTH WEIGHT LOSS PLAN – base number

	Under 205	206-280	281-320	321-380	381+
Age 10-26	10	9	8	7	6
Age 27-42	9	8	7	6	5
Age 43+	8	7	6	5	5

MEN

1+ YEAR WEIGHT LOSS PLAN – base number

	Under 205	206-280	281-320	321-386	387+
Age 10-26	11	10	9	8	7
Age 27-42	10	9	8	7	6
Age 43+	9	8	7	6	5

Revolving Daily Calorie Maximums

Using your base number, current weight, and activity level, locate your revolving daily Calorie maximums on the following charts.

R.L. Erickson C.H.P.

Base Number 11

Base 11
Wt. 110-138

Activity	Day 1	Day 2	Day 3	Day 4	Day 5	Day 6	Day 7
Inactive	840	1100	1235	1340	1435	1490	1655
Average	940	1200	1335	1430	1535	1590	1755
Active	1140	1400	1535	1640	1735	1790	1955

Base 11
Wt. 139-174

Activity	Day 1	Day 2	Day 3	Day 4	Day 5	Day 6	Day 7
Inactive	1100	1440	1615	1785	1910	1960	2130
Average	1200	1540	1715	1885	2010	2060	2230
Active	1400	1740	1915	2085	2210	2260	2430

Base 11
Wt. 175-210

Activity	Day 1	Day 2	Day 3	Day 4	Day 5	Day 6	Day 7
Inactive	1360	1785	1995	2205	2380	2420	2630
Average	1460	1885	2095	2305	2480	2520	2730
Active	1660	2085	2395	2505	2680	2720	2930

Base Number 10

Base 10
Wt. 110- 152

Activity	Day 1	Day 2	Day 3	Day 4	Day 5	Day 6	Day 7
Inactive	840	1100	1235	1340	1435	1490	1655
Average	940	1200	1335	1430	1535	1590	1755
Active	1140	1400	1535	1640	1735	1790	1955

Base 10
Wt. 153-192

Activity	Day 1	Day 2	Day 3	Day 4	Day 5	Day 6	Day 7
Inactive	1100	1440	1615	1785	1910	1960	2130
Average	1200	1540	1715	1885	2010	2060	2230
Active	1400	1740	1915	2085	2210	2260	2430

Base 10
Wt. 193-232

Activity	Day 1	Day 2	Day 3	Day 4	Day 5	Day 6	Day 7
Inactive	1360	1785	1995	2205	2380	2420	2630
Average	1460	1885	2095	2305	2480	2520	2730
Active	1660	2085	2395	2505	2680	2720	2930

Base 10
Wt. 233-272

Activity	Day 1	Day 2	Day 3	Day 4	Day 5	Day 6	Day 7
Inactive	1620	2120	2375	2630	2820	2880	3130
Average	1720	1820	2475	2730	2920	2980	3230
Active	1920	2420	2675	2930	3120	3180	3430

Base 10
Wt. 273-280

Activity	Day 1	Day 2	Day 3	Day 4	Day 5	Day 6	Day 7
Inactive	1880	2465	2755	3045	3275	3340	3630
Average	1980	2565	2855	3145	3375	3440	3730
Active	2180	2865	3055	3345	3575	3640	3930

R.L. Erickson C.H.P.

Base Number 9

Base 9
Wt. 110-125

Activity	Day 1	Day 2	Day 3	Day 4	Day 5	Day 6	Day 7
Inactive	580	760	855	945	995	1035	1130
Average	680	860	955	1045	1095	1135	1230
Active	880	1060	1185	1245	1295	1335	1530

Base 9
Wt. 126-169

Activity	Day 1	Day 2	Day 3	Day 4	Day 5	Day 6	Day 7
Inactive	840	1100	1235	1340	1435	1490	1655
Average	940	1200	1335	1430	1535	1590	1755
Active	1140	1400	1535	1640	1735	1790	1955

Base 9
Wt. 170-213

Activity	Day 1	Day 2	Day 3	Day 4	Day 5	Day 6	Day 7
Inactive	1100	1440	1615	1785	1910	1960	2130
Average	1200	1540	1715	1885	2010	2060	2230
Active	1400	1740	1915	2085	2210	2260	2430

Base 9
Wt. 214- 257

Activity	Day 1	Day 2	Day 3	Day 4	Day 5	Day 6	Day 7
Inactive	1360	1785	1995	2205	2380	2420	2630
Average	1460	1885	2095	2305	2480	2520	2730
Active	1660	2085	2395	2505	2680	2720	2930

Base 9
Wt. 258-302

Activity	Day 1	Day 2	Day 3	Day 4	Day 5	Day 6	Day 7
Inactive	1620	2120	2375	2630	2820	2880	3130
Average	1720	1820	2475	2730	2920	2980	3230
Active	1920	2420	2675	2930	3120	3180	3430

Base 9
Wt. 303-320

Activity	Day 1	Day 2	Day 3	Day 4	Day 5	Day 6	Day 7
Inactive	1880	2465	2755	3045	3275	3340	3630
Average	1980	2565	2855	3145	3375	3440	3730
Active	2180	2865	3055	3345	3575	3640	3930

R.L. Erickson C.H.P.

Base Number 8

Base 8
Wt. 120-140

Activity	Day 1	Day 2	Day 3	Day 4	Day 5	Day 6	Day 7
Inactive	**580**	760	855	945	995	1035	1130
Average	**680**	860	955	1045	1095	1135	1230
Active	**880**	1060	1185	1245	1295	1335	1530

Base 8
Wt. 141-191

Activity	Day 1	Day 2	Day 3	Day 4	Day 5	Day 6	Day 7
Inactive	**840**	1100	1235	1340	1435	1490	1655
Average	940	1200	1335	1430	1535	1590	1755
Active	1140	1400	1535	1640	1735	1790	1955

Base 8
Wt. 192-240

Activity	Day 1	Day 2	Day 3	Day 4	Day 5	Day 6	Day 7
Inactive	**1100**	1440	1615	1785	1910	1960	2130
Average	**1200**	1540	1715	1885	2010	2060	2230
Active	**1400**	1740	1915	2085	2210	2260	2430

Base 8
Wt. 241-290

Activity	Day 1	Day 2	Day 3	Day 4	Day 5	Day 6	Day 7
Inactive	1360	1785	1995	2205	2380	2420	2630
Average	1460	1885	2095	2305	2480	2520	2730
Active	1660	2085	2395	2505	2680	2720	2930

Base 8
Wt. 291-340

Activity	Day 1	Day 2	Day 3	Day 4	Day 5	Day 6	Day 7
Inactive	1620	2120	2375	2630	2820	2880	3130
Average	1720	1820	2475	2730	2920	2980	3230
Active	1920	2420	2675	2930	3120	3180	3430

Base 8
Wt. 341-386

Activity	Day 1	Day 2	Day 3	Day 4	Day 5	Day 6	Day 7
Inactive	1880	2465	2755	3045	3275	3340	3630
Average	1980	2565	2855	3145	3375	3440	3730
Active	2180	2865	3055	3345	3575	3640	3930

R.L. Erickson C.H.P.

Base Number 7

Base 7
Wt. 110-160

Activity	Day 1	Day 2	Day 3	Day 4	Day 5	Day 6	Day 7
Inactive	580	760	855	945	995	1035	1130
Average	680	860	955	1045	1095	1135	1230
Active	880	1060	1185	1245	1295	1335	1530

Base7
Wt. 161-217

Activity	Day 1	Day 2	Day 3	Day 4	Day 5	Day 6	Day 7
Inactive	840	1100	1235	1340	1435	1490	1655
Average	940	1200	1335	1430	1535	1590	1755
Active	1140	1400	1535	1640	1735	1790	1955

Base 7
Wt. 218-274

Activity	Day 1	Day 2	Day 3	Day 4	Day 5	Day 6	Day 7
Inactive	1100	1440	1615	1785	1910	1960	2130
Average	1200	1540	1715	1885	2010	2060	2230
Active	1400	1740	1915	2085	2210	2260	2430

Base 7
Wt. 275-331

Activity	Day 1	Day 2	Day 3	Day 4	Day 5	Day 6	Day 7
Inactive	1360	1785	1995	2205	2380	2420	2630
Average	1460	1885	2095	2305	2480	2520	2730
Active	1660	2085	2395	2505	2680	2720	2930

Base 7
Wt. 332-386

Activity	Day 1	Day 2	Day 3	Day 4	Day 5	Day 6	Day 7
Inactive	1620	2120	2375	2630	2820	2880	3130
Average	1720	1820	2475	2730	2920	2980	3230
Active	1920	2420	2675	2930	3120	3180	3430

Base 7
Wt. 387-+

Activity	Day 1	Day 2	Day 3	Day 4	Day 5	Day 6	Day 7
Inactive	1880	2465	2755	3045	3275	3340	3630
Average	1980	2565	2855	3145	3375	3440	3730
Active	2180	2865	3055	3345	3575	3640	3930

R.L. Erickson C.H.P.

Base Number 6

Base 6
Wt. 201-253

Activity	Day 1	Day 2	Day 3	Day 4	Day 5	Day 6	Day 7
Inactive	840	1100	1235	1340	1435	1490	1655
Average	940	1200	1335	1430	1535	1590	1755
Active	1140	1400	1535	1640	1735	1790	1955

Base 6
Wt. 254-320

Activity	Day 1	Day 2	Day 3	Day 4	Day 5	Day 6	Day 7
Inactive	1100	1440	1615	1785	1910	1960	2130
Average	1200	1540	1715	1885	2010	2060	2230
Active	1400	1740	1915	2085	2210	2260	2430

Base 6
Wt. 321-386

Activity	Day 1	Day 2	Day 3	Day 4	Day 5	Day 6	Day 7
Inactive	1360	1785	1995	2205	2380	2420	2630
Average	1460	1885	2095	2305	2480	2520	2730
Active	1660	2085	2395	2505	2680	2720	2930

Base 6
Wt. 387-+

Activity	Day 1	Day 2	Day 3	Day 4	Day 5	Day 6	Day 7
Inactive	1620	2120	2375	2630	2820	2880	3130
Average	1720	1820	2475	2730	2920	2980	3230
Active	1920	2420	2675	2930	3120	3180	3430

Base Number 5

Base 5
Wt. 188-253

Activity	Day 1	Day 2	Day 3	Day 4	Day 5	Day 6	Day 7
Inactive	840	1100	1235	1340	1435	1490	1655
Average	940	1200	1335	1430	1535	1590	1755
Active	1140	1400	1535	1640	1735	1790	1955

Base 5
Wt. 254-320

Activity	Day 1	Day 2	Day 3	Day 4	Day 5	Day 6	Day 7
Inactive	1100	1440	1615	1785	1910	1960	2130
Average	1200	1540	1715	1885	2010	2060	2230
Active	1400	1740	1915	2085	2210	2260	2430

Base 5
Wt. 321-386

Activity	Day 1	Day 2	Day 3	Day 4	Day 5	Day 6	Day 7
Inactive	1360	1785	1995	2205	2380	2420	2630
Average	1460	1885	2095	2305	2480	2520	2730
Active	1660	2085	2395	2505	2680	2720	2930

Base 5
Wt. 387-+

Activity	Day 1	Day 2	Day 3	Day 4	Day 5	Day 6	Day 7
Inactive	1620	2120	2375	2630	2820	2880	3130
Average	1720	1820	2475	2730	2920	2980	3230
Active	1920	2420	2675	2930	3120	3180	3430

Calorie Charts

By now you should realize that "it isn't what you eat but rather the amount of calories consumed within your daily calorie maximum each day that counts." With this statement in mind, I developed this unique calorie chart.

The majority of daily calorie charts merely list foods in alphabetical order or by foods groups and use the standard USDA Nutrient database. It is hard to use these calorie counters, as many times you need a calculator to figure out the calories contained in the foods you are eating.

Since the average weekly calorie maximums for weight loss are usually less than 2000 calories per day, and most people eat a minimum of three to seven times per day (meals plus snacking), a calorie chart should reflect the food groups in calorie portion amounts, at acceptable calorie amounts. If a particular meal or food is, for example, 1500 calories per serving, it may be unacceptable even if your daily maximum is 3000 calories.

This chart is therefore calculated in 100- and 200-calorie intervals up to 700 calories per serving. Foods groups exceeding 700 calories per serving are grouped in a separate "Cautionary" category. If you must eat these foods, you may do so; but it is recommended just not at one sitting.

Also, when reading labels of combined or packaged foods, i.e., soups, chips, crackers, etc., be sure you understand the serving size. Calories, unless otherwise stipulated, are always listed in serving size and a package or can may contain several servings. By eating a whole can of soup or bag of chips, you could be eating 2 to 15 times the listed calorie amount.

Finally, food is grouped into 18 subcategories and when determining the amount of food you are consuming, it is important to know just how restaurants, fast food, and the food industry lists foods – by weight or volume.

The following food group and conversion charts may be helpful in making an informed decision on whether to eat certain foods.

Food sub-groups:
Protein-P, Carbohydrate-C, Fats-F

- **Meat— beef, lamb, pork, wild meats—P-F**
- **Poultry— chicken, turkey, wild fowl— P-F**
- **Fish— all fresh and saltwater fish and shellfish P-F**
- **Eggs— chicken, duck, geese——P-F**
- **Dry Beans— all beans and peas— P-F-C**
- **Nuts— peanut, walnuts, cashews—— P-F-C**
- **Fruits—apples, all berries, bananas, citrus, juices etc. — C**
- **Vegetables— all green, yellow, red, potato, yams—— C**
- **Milk— skim, whole, cottage cheese, ice cream— P-F**
- **Yogurt— non-fat, frozen, low fat, regular—— P-F**
- **Cheese— hard and soft ——P-F**
- **Fats— butter, margarine, mayonnaise, sour cream, —— F**
- **Oils— salad dressing—— F**
- **Sweets— chocolate bars, candies———— P-F-C**
- **Bread— biscuits, breads, rolls, pancakes, Danish cakes, cookies, tortilla, croissant, donuts- C-F**
- **Cereal— breakfast types ———C-F**
- **Rice— white, brown ———P-F-C**
- **Pasta— spaghetti, pastas— C-F**

All foods, whether engineered or naturally prepared, *candy—fast food—canned food—restaurant—homemade—snack food—frozen food—deli—health food—beverages* are made from these 18 sub-groups; 11 are protein-based, 5 are carbohydrate-based, and 14 contain fats. Foods contain the other nutrients such as water, vitamins, and minerals in varying amounts, but digestion is used to breaks down food to just these four components:

- **Amino acids** from proteins
- **Sugar** from carbohydrates
- **Fatty acids** from fats
- **Glycerol** from fats

CONVERSION CHART

These conversion amounts will allow you to easily compute the amounts of calories in the food you enjoy. For example, if you love milk and drink ½ gallon a day, with one cup of milk being 150 calories, that is 8 cups x 150 calories = 1200 calories you will consume. Or a fast food sandwich is 800 calories that weighs 238 g, or about 8.2 ounces, so it has about 100 calories per ounce.

Ounces to Grams

1 oz. = 28.35 g
2 oz. = 56.70g
3 oz. = 85.05 g
4 oz. = 113.40 g
6 oz. = 170.10 g
8 oz. = 226.80 g
12 oz. = 340.20 g
16 oz. (1lb.) = 453.60 g

Ounces to Dry Measurement

3 teaspoons = 1 tablespoon
2 tablespoons = 1 oz
4 oz. flour = 125 g = 1 cup
4 oz. oatmeal = 124 g = 1 cup (scant)
4 oz. butter and other fats, including cheese = 125 g = 1 stick
8 oz. butter and other fats, including cheese = 250 g = 1 cup
7 oz. caster/granulated sugar = 200 g = 1 cup
8 oz. caster/granulated sugar = 250 g = 1¼ cups
8 oz. meat (chopped/minced/ground) = 250 g = 1 cup

Ounces to liquid measurement
1 tablespoon liquid = 15 ml
16 tablespoons = 8 fluid ounces = 100 ml = 1 cup
8 fluid ounces = 250 ml = 1 cup = ½ pint
16 fluid ounces = 500 ml = 2 cups = 1 pint
2 pints = 4 cups = 1 quart
2 quarts = 8 cups = 4 pints = ½ gallon
4 quarts = 16 cups= 8 pints =1 gallons

The New Calorie Counter

Assorted fast foods and the 18 food sub-groups

R.L. Erickson C.H.P.

Calories: 0-99

Fast foods

Type/Serving Size	Calories	Type/Serving Size	Calories
Boston Market Broccoli with red peppers 3.4 oz.	60	**Subway** Veggie Delite salad 3 oz.	60
Denny's Green beans with bacon 4 oz.	60	**Dairy Queen** Vanilla Orange Bar 2.3 oz.	60
Denny's Chicken Noodle Soup 8 oz.	60	**Arby's** Scrambled egg one	70
Hardees Mashed potatoes, small 113 g	70	**Boston Market** Fruit salad 6 oz.	75
Boston Market Fruit salad 5.5 oz.	70	**Long John Silver's** Corn Cobbette 3 oz.	80
Schlotzsky's French Onion Soup 227 grams	78	**Panda Express** Egg Flower Soup, 12 oz.	80
Denny's Carrots in honey glaze 4 oz.	80	**Schlotzsky's** Minestrone soup 227 g	89
Boston Market Green Beans 3.0 oz.	80		

Eggs

Type/Serving Size	Calories	Type/Serving Size	Calories
Egg Boiled One	75	**Egg** Poached One	75

171

Calories 0-99

Fruits

Type/Serving Size	Calories	Type/Serving Size	Calories
Apple 1 medium	80	**Apricots,** dried 4 halves	40
Apricots, fresh 1 medium	20	**Avocado** ¼ medium	80
Blackberries 1 cup	75	**Blueberries** 1 cup	80
Cantaloupe 1 cup	55	**Cherries,** maraschino 10 medium	99
Cherries, sour, fresh 1 cup	80	**Cranberries,** fresh 1 cup	50
Grapefruit 1 medium	80	**Grapes** 25 medium	88
Honeydew melon 1 cup	60	**Kiwi** 1 medium	45
Mandarin oranges 1 cup	99	**Nectarine** 1 medium	65
Orange 1 medium	60	**Peach** 1 medium	40
Pear 1 medium	99	**Pineapple, fresh** 1 cup	75
Plums, fresh 2 medium	70	**Plums,** dried 5 medium	99
Raspberries 1 cup	60	**Strawberries** 1 cup	50
Tangerine 1 medium	35	**Watermelon** 1 cup	50

172

Calories 0-99

Vegetables, cooked* and raw

Type/Serving Size	Calories	Type/Serving Size	Calories
Artichokes* 1 medium	60	**Asparagus*,** 2 cups	80
Broccoli* 2 cups	80	**Broccoli,** raw 2 cups	20
Brussels sprouts* 1 cup	60	**Beets** canned or cooked 1 cup	55
Cabbage* 2 cups	60	**Cabbage** Raw 2 cups	30
Carrots*, 1 cup	70	**Carrots,** raw 1 large	30
Catsup 1 tablespoon	15	**Cauliflower*** 1 cup	35
Celery, raw 1 stalk	5	**Collard greens*** 1 cup	25
Corn grits* Plain instant 1 packet	80	**Corn on the cob*** 1 ear	80
Cucumber, raw 1 medium	40	**Green beans*** 1 cup	50
Lettuce, raw 2 cups	10	**Mushrooms,** canned 1 cup	40
Mushrooms, raw 2 cup	40	**Onions,** raw 1 cup	60
Pea pods* 1 cup	70	**Peppers,** sweet, raw 1 cup	40
Potato, french-fries, homemade 10 medium	99	**Pumpkin** 1 cup	50

Calories 0-99

Vegetables, cooked* and raw

Type/Serving Size	Calories	Type/Serving Size	Calories
Spinach* 1 cup	40	**Spinach,** raw 2 cups	20
Squash 1 cup	99	**Tomatoes,** canned 1 cup	50
Tomatoes, raw **1 medium**	25	**Turnip** 1 cup	55
Zucchini 1 cup	40		

Fats and Oils

Type/Serving Size	Calories	Type/Serving Size	Calories
Cooking spray 4-second spray	20	**Cream,** whipping 1 tablespoon	50
Half and half, regular 1 tablespoon	20	**Half and half,** fat-free 1 tablespoon	10
Mayonnaise, Low-fat 2 tablespoons	70	**Mayonnaise,** fat-free 2 tablespoons	20
Sour cream, Regular 2 tablespoons	60	**Sour cream,** reduced-fat 2 tablespoons	40

Breads and snacks

Type/Serving Size	Calories	Type/Serving Size	Calories
Bread, white/wheat 1 slice	80	**Bread,** light 1slice	40
Melba toast 4 pieces	80	**Dinner Roll,** 1 medium	85
Croutons ½ cup	90	**Animal crackers** 6 plain	85

Calories 0-99

Breads and snacks

Type/Serving Size	Calories	Type/Serving Size	Calories
Butter crackers 6 crackers	96	**Oyster crackers** 30 crackers	80
Saltines 8 crackers	96	**Popcorn,** Air popped 3 cups	90
Popcorn, Microwave 3 cups	99	**Popcorn,** Microwave light 3 cups	60
Bran flakes ¾ cup	99	**Puffed rice** 1 cup	50

Beverages

Type/Serving Size	Calories	Type/Serving Size	Calories
All diet cola 12 oz.	0-1	**Beer – Lager, generic** 12 oz.	96
Beer - Brown Ale 12 oz.	96	**Beer - Amstel Light** 12 oz.	96
Beer - Miller Lite 12 oz.	95	**Spirits** Apricot brandy 1shot (1oz.)	80

R.L. Erickson C.H.P.

Calories 100-300

Assorted fast foods and the 18 food sub-groups

R.L. Erickson C.H.P.

Calories: 100-300

Fast Foods

Type/Serving Size	Calories	Type/Serving Size	Calories
Schlotzsky's Tomato Florentine Soup, 227 g	100	**Subway** Turkey Breast Salad 290 g	105
Schlotzsky's Vegetable Beef Barley Soup 227 g	100	**Pizza Hut** The Edge The Works 1 square, 63 g	110
McDonald's Grilled Chicken Caesar Salad 163 g	100	**Wendy's** Deluxe Garden Salad 270 g	110
McDonald's Garden Salad 149 g	100	**Wendy's** Caesar Side Salad 92 g	110
Domino's Sweet Icing 1 oz.	103	**Subway** Ham Salad 289 g	112
Subway Peach Pizzazz (Fuizie Express, small) 341 g	103	**Subway** Berry Lishus (Fuizle Express, small) 369 g	113
Subway Roast Beef Salad 290 g	114	**Wendy's** Hidden Valley® Ranch red, reduced fat (1 packet) 57 g	120
Subway Turkey Breast & Ham Salad 299 g	117	**Kentucky Fried Chicken** Mashed Potato w/ gravy 136 g	120
Domino's Breadsticks 1 piece, 37.2 g	117	**Schlotzsky's** Chicken Noodle Old-Fashioned Soup 227 g	122
Domino's CinnaStix 1 stick, 32.05 g	123	**McDonald's** 1000 Island Dressing 1 package, 44.4 ml	130
Subway Sunrise Refresher (Fuizle Express - small) 341 g	119-137	**McDonald's** Red French Dressing reduced calorie 1 package, 44.4 ml	130

Calories: 100-300

Fast Foods

Type/Serving Size	Calories	Type/Serving Size	Calories
McDonald's hash browns 53 g	130	**Kentucky Fried Chicken** Original Recipe Chicken Wings 1 wing, 47 g	140
Pizza Hut Bread Stick (1 serving) 38 g	130	**Kentucky Fried Chicken** Original Recipe Chicken Drumstick, 61 g	140
Wendy's Soft Bread Sticks 44 g	130	**Papa John's** Bread Sticks 1/8 order (1 stick) 55 g	140
Boston Market Green Bean Casserole 6.0 oz.	130	**Domino's** Cheesy Bread 1 piece, 43.1 g	142
Subway Roasted Chicken Breast Salad 304 g	137	**Subway** Subway Club Salad 323 g	145
Arby's BBQ Vinaigrette Dressing 1 package, 2 oz.	140	**Schlotzsky's** 7 Bean Medley Soup 227 g	145
Kentucky Fried Chicken corn on the cob 162 g	150	**McDonald's** English Muffin 57 g	150
McDonald's Chef Salad 206 g	150	**McDonald's** Vanilla Ice Cream Cone reduced fat 90 g	150
McDonald's Caesar Dressing 1 package, 44.4 ml	150	**Pizza Hut** Garlic Bread 1 slice, 37 g	150
Taco Bell Cinnamon Twists 1.25 oz.	150	**Arby's** Roast Chicken Salad 420 g	160
Burger King Chicken Caesar Salad (no dressing or croutons) 257 g	160	**Pizza Hut** Thin'n'Crispy Pizza w/Ham (medium pizza) 1 slice, 82 g	170

Calories: 100-300

Fast Foods

Type/Serving Size	Calories	Type/Serving Size	Calories
McDonald's Honey Mustard Dressing 1 package, 44.4 ml	**160**	**McDonald's** Ranch Dressing 1 package, 44.4 ml	**170**
McDonald's Scrambled Eggs 2 eggs, 102 g	**160**	**Taco Bell** Taco 2.75 oz.	**170**
Pizza Hut The Edge, Meat Lover's Pizza 1 square, 58 g	**160**	**Kentucky Fried Chicken** Hot & Spicy Chicken - Drumstick 64 g	**175**
Wendy's Frosty Dairy Dessert Junior 113 g	**170**	**Kentucky Fried Chicken** Biscuit 1 biscuit, 56 g	**180**
Burger King Chicken Tenders - 4 pieces 62 g	**170**	**Kentucky Fried Chicken** Macaroni & Cheese 153 g	**180**
McDonald's Sausage 1 sausage, 43 g	**170**	**Papa John's** Cheese Sticks 1/7 order 2 sticks, 60 g	**180**
Taco Bell Pintos 'n' Cheese 4.5 oz.	**180**	**Subway** Steak & Cheese Salad 315 g	**182**
Boston Market Rice Pilaf 5.1 oz.	**180**	**Kentucky Fried Chicken** BBQ Baked Beans 156 g	**190**
Burger King Onion Rings small 51 g	**180**	**Pizza Hut** Thin'n' Crispy Pepperoni Pizza (medium) 1 slice, 81 g	**190**
Pizza Hut Thin'n' Crispy Veggie Lover's Pizza (medium) 1 slice, 115 g	**190**	**Taco Bell** Soft Taco chicken or steak 3.5 oz.	**190**

Taco Bell
Mexican Rice   **190**
4.75 oz.

Wendy's
Crispy Chicken Nuggets   **190**
(4 piece Kids' Meal)
60 g

Calories: 100-300

Fast Foods

Type/Serving Size	Calories	Type/Serving Size	Calories
Boston Market Coyote Bean Salad 5.3 oz.	**190**	**Denny's** Cream of Broccoli Soup 8 oz.	**193**
Subway Ham (Deli Sandwich) 147 g	**194**	**Subway** Oatmeal Raisin Cookie 48 g	**197**
Kentucky Fried Chicken Extra Crispy Chicken - Drumstick 67 g	**195**	**Subway** Seafood & Crab Salad 314 g	**198**
Pizza Hut Mild Buffalo Wings 5 pieces, 84 g	**200**	**Boston Market** Corn Bread, 2.4 oz.	**200**
Pizza Hut Thin'n' Crispy w/Cheese (medium pizza) 1 slice 85 g	**200**	**Wendy's** Grilled Chicken Salad 344 g	**200**
Pizza Hut Thin'n' Crispy w/Chicken Supreme (medium pizza) 1 slice 113 g	**200**	**Kentucky Fried Chicken** Little Bucket Parfait Strawberry Shortcake 99 g	**200**
Subway 6" Veggie Delite Sub 163 g	**200**	**Subway** Subway Melt Salad 318 g	**203**
Subway Turkey Breast (Deli Sandwich) 157 g	**200**	**Subway** Roast Beef (Deli Sandwich) 157 g	**206**
Wendy's Hidden Valley Ranch Dressing (1pkt) 57 g	**200**	**Subway** Cookie – M & M choc chip/ chunk Peanut, sugar, Macadamia — 48 g	**209-222**
Arby's Grilled Chicken Salad 464 g	**210**	**Pizza Hut** Hot Buffalo Wings (4 pieces) 87 g	**210**

Calories: 100-300

Fast Foods

Type/Serving Size	Calories	Type/Serving Size	Calories
Burger King Chicken Tenders - 5 pieces 77 g	210	**Taco Bell** Soft Taco – Beef 3.5 oz.	210
Kentucky Fried Chicken Hot & Spicy Chicken – Whole Wing 55 g	210	**Wendy's** Taco Chips 42 g	210
McDonald's French Fries Small 68 g	210	**Wendy's** Chili – Small 227 g	210
Schlotzsky's Timberline Chili Soup 227 g	210	**McDonald's** McDonaldland Cookies (1 bag) 57 g	230
Arby's Home Style Fries (Child-Size) 85 g	220	**Pizza Hut** Hand Tossed Chicken Supreme (medium pizza) 1 slice 124 g	230
Pizza Hut Hand Tossed Veggie Lover's (medium pizza) 1 slice 126 g	220	**Wendy's** Italian Caesar Dressing (1pkt) 43 g	230
Kentucky Fried Chicken Extra Crispy Chicken – Whole Wing 55 g	220	**Kentucky Fried Chicken** Cole Slaw 142 g	232
Papa John's Thin Crust Pizza – Garden Special (large 14") 1/8 124 g	226	**Papa John's** Thin Crust Pizza w/ Cheese (14" large) 1/8 95 g	233
Arby's Grilled Chicken Caesar Salad (Fresh) 338 g	230	**Schlotzsky's** Boston Clam Chowder 243 g	233

Calories: 100-300

Fast Foods

Type/Serving Size	Calories	Type/Serving Size	Calories
Burger King French Fries – Small (salted) 74 g	230	**Subway** Tuna Salad 314 g	238
Burger King Hash Brown Rounds – Small Serving Size: 75 g	230	**McDonald's** Biscuit 69 g	240
Kentucky Fried Chicken Potato Salad 160 g	230	**Pizza Hut** Hand Tossed w/ Cheese (medium pizza) 1 slice 106 g	240
Arby's Grilled Chicken Caesar Salad (Fresh) 338 g	230	**Taco Bell** Soft Taco Supreme- Chicken or steak 4.75 oz.	240
Boston Market Broccoli Rice Casserole 6.0 oz.	240	**Wendy's** French Dressing (1pkt) 57 g	250
Arby's Potato Cakes (2) 100 g	250	**Pizza Hut** thin'n crispy w/ Pepperoni Lover's (medium pizza) 1 slice 97 g	250
Burger King Chicken Tenders - 6 pieces 92 g	250	**Pizza Hut** Apple Dessert Pizza 81 g	250
Kentucky Fried Chicken Original Recipe Chicken- Thigh 91 g	250	**Subway** 6" Turkey Breast Sub 220 g	254
Pizza Hut Hand Tossed Pepperoni Lover's (Medium pizza) 1 slice 106 g	250	**Pizza Hut** Sicilian w/ Ham (medium pizza) 1 slice108 g	257
Pizza Hut thin'n crispy w/ Pepperoni Lover's (medium pizza) 1 slice 97 g	250	**Arby's** Light Roast Chicken Deluxe Sandwich 194 g	260

Calories: 100-300

Fast Foods

Type/Serving Size	Calories	Type/Serving Size	Calories
Pizza Hut Cherry Dessert Pizza 81 g	250	**Arby's** Light Roast Turkey Deluxe Sandwich 194 g	260
Pizza Hut thin'n crispy w/ Pepperoni Lover's (medium pizza) 1 slice 97 g	250	**McDonald's** Baked Apple Pie 77 g	260
Pizza Hut thin'n crispy w/ Supreme (medium pizza) 1 slice 117 g	250	**Pizza Hut** Hand Tossed w/ Ham (medium pizza) 1 slice 118 g	260
Taco Bell Tostada 6.25 oz.	250	**Wendy's** Thousand Island Dressing (1 pkt) 57 g	260
Boston Market Red Beans and Rice 8.0 oz.	260	**Pizza Hut** Pan Pizza Veggie Lover's (medium pizza) 1 slice 130 g	270
Taco Bell Soft Taco Supreme - Beef 5 oz.	260	**Pizza Hut** Sicilian Veggie Lover's (medium pizza) 1 slice 132 g	270
Subway 6" Ham Sub 219 g	261	**Pizza Hut** Pan Pizza Chicken Supreme (medium pizza) 1 slice 128 g	270
Subway 6" Roast Beef Sub 220 g	264	**Pizza Hut** thin'n crispy W/ Pork or beef Topping (Medium pizza) 1 slice 106 g	270
Papa John's Thin Crust Pizza w/ Pepperoni(large 14") 1/8 98 g	266	**Wendy's** Jr. Hamburger 117 g	270

Calories: 100-300

Fast Foods

Type/Serving Size	Calories	Type/Serving Size	Calories
Subway 6" Turkey Breast & Ham Sub 229 g	267	**Wendy's** Kids' Meal Fries 91 g	270
Burger King Chicken Whooper Jr. (w/o Mayo) 155 g	270	**Subway** BMT Salad 312 g	273
Pizza Hut Hand Tossed Supreme (medium pizza) 1 slice 129 g	270	**Subway** 6" Honey Mustard Turkey w/ Cucumber 232 g	275
Kentucky Fried Chicken Hot & Spicy Chicken – Whole Wing 55 g	210	**Arby's** Biscuit w/ butter 82 g	280
Pizza Hut Sicilian Chicken Supreme (medium pizza) 1 slice 130 g	270	**Arby's** Light Grilled Chicken Sandwich 174 g	280
Kentucky Fried Chicken Potato Wedges 135 g	280	**Papa John's** Original Crust Pizza w/ Cheese (large 14") 1/8 131 g	283
Kentucky Fried Chicken Colonels Pies – Strawberry Crème Pie 1 Slice, 78 g	280	**Kentucky Fried Chicken** Little Bucket Parfait - Chocolate Cream 113 g	290
McDonald's Hamburger 107 g	280	**Arby's** Honey French Dressing (1 pkg) 2 oz.	290
McDonald's Chocolate Chip Cookies 1 bag, 56 g	280	**McDonald's** Strawberry Sundae 178 g	290
McDonald's Fruit 'n Yogurt Parfait (w/o granola) 310 g	280	**McDonald's** Sausage Breakfast Burrito 113 g	290

Calories: 100-300

Fast Foods

Type/Serving Size	Calories	Type/Serving Size	Calories
Papa John's		**Pizza Hut**	
Original Crust Pizza Garden Special (large 14") 1/8 152 g	280	Hand Tossed Super Supreme (medium pizza) 1 slice 139 g	290
Pizza Hut Pan Pizza or Sicilian w/ Pepperoni (medium pizza) 1 slice 106 g	280	**Pizza Hut** Hand Tossed Super Supreme (medium pizza) 1 slice 139 g	290
Pizza Hut thin'n crispy w/ Super Supreme (medium pizza) 1 slice 130 g	280	**Subway** Western Egg or ham & egg (Breakfast Sandwich) 167 g	290
Boston Market Macaroni and Cheese 6.8 oz.	280	**Taco Bell** MexiMelt 4.75 oz.	290
Papa John's Thin Crust Pizza w/ Sausage (large 14") 1/8 109 g	283	**Taco Bell** Gordita Nacho Cheese – Chicken or Steak 5.5 oz.	290
Subway 6" Subway Club Sub 253 g	294	**McDonald's** Egg McMuffin 138 g	300
Arby's Homestyle Fries (Small) 113 g	300	**McDonald's** Chicken McGrill Sandwich (plain w/o mayo) 199 g	300
Kentucky Fried Chicken Colonels Crispy Strips (3) 115 g	300	**Taco Bell** Gordita Supreme - Chicken –Steak or Beef 5.5 oz.	300
McDonald's Lowfat Apple Bran Muffin 114 g	300	**Wendy's** Grilled Chicken Sandwich 188 g	300
Boston Market Cole Slaw 6.5 oz.	300		

Calories 100-300
Candies

Type/Serving Size	Calories	Type/Serving Size	Calories
York		**D.L. Clark**	
Peppermint Patty	170	Clark Bar	240
1 medium patty		1 medium bar	
Hershey		**Reese's**	
Almond Joy	180	Reese's Cup	240
1 medium bar		1 medium package	
Nestle		**Reese's**	
100 Grand	200	Nut Rageous	250
1 medium bar		1 medium bar	
Leaf		**M&M/Mars**	
Heath Bar	210	Musketeers	260
1 medium bar		1 medium bar	
Nestle		**M&M/Mars**	
Milk Chocolate	200	Twix	280
1 medium bar		1 medium bar	
Reese's		**Hershey**	
Kit Kat	220	Mr. Good Bar	280
1 medium panel		1 medium bar	
Hershey –		**Hershey**	
Rolo	230	5th Avenue	280
1 medium bar		1 medium bar	
Hershey		**M&M/Mars**	
Chocolate Bar	230	Snickers	280
1 medium bar		1 medium bar	
Nestle		**M&M/Mars**	
Butterfinger	200	Milky Way	280
1 medium bar		1 medium bar	
Hershey			
Chocolate w/Almond	230		
1 medium bar			

Calories 100-300
Meats

Processed and Deli Meats— alphabetical

Type/Serving Size	Calories	Type/Serving Size	Calories
Bacon, Fried 6 slices, (20 slices per-lb.)	**210**	**Hot dog** 1small —1.6 oz.	**145**
Beef jerky (3 strips) 3 oz.	**270**	**Pepperoni** (3 avg. slices) 2 oz.	**280**
Bologna (4 avg. slices) 3 oz.	**270**	**Roast beef**, deli (1slice ¾" thick) ½ lb	**240**
Canadian bacon (4 avg. slices) 3 oz.	**135**	**Sausage**, Italian (1 slice ¼" thick) 1—2 oz.	**215**
Ham, deli (4 avg. slices) 3 oz.	**120**	**Sausage,** Polish (1 med.) 1— 2.7 oz.	**240**
		Sausage, smoked (Med.) 1—2 oz.	**190**

Poultry: Homemade cooked

Type/Serving Size	Calories	Type/Serving Size	Calories
Chicken breast w/skin (1large breast) 5 oz.	**285**	**Turkey breast,** Deli 10 ounce (14-16slices)	**300**
Chicken breast, **no skin** (1large breast) 5 oz.	**233**	**Turkey,** Dark meat, skin 4 oz. (1/2 thigh)	**247**
Chicken breast, deli (7-8 slices) 5 ounce	**225**	**Turkey,** Light meat, skin (1/2 breast) 6 oz.	**280**
Chicken thighs, no skin (1med.) 5 oz.	**275**	**Turkey,** Light meat, no skin (1/6 breast) 6 oz.	**240**
Chicken thighs, skin (1med.) 4 oz.	**280**	**Turkey Ground, lean** 5 oz. (2/3 cup)	**283**
Chicken wings, Roasted 3 (no sauce)	**300**	**Turkey Ground,** Extra-lean 6 oz. (3/4 cup)	**240**

190

Calories 100-300
Fish and Seafood Homemade cooked

Type/Serving Size	Calories	Type/Serving Size	Calories
Catfish Baked 6 oz.	260	**Crab**, Blue fresh ½ lb	240
Clams 18 large	270	**Crab**, Blue canned 2 cup	280
Cod ½ lb	240	**Crab**, Imitation ½ LB	240
Halibut, Atlantic 6 oz. (4x4x¼")	240	**Mussels** 6 oz. (10 shells)	290
Lobster (1med tail) ½ lb.	293	**Orange Roughy** Baked (1-2 avg. fillets) 12 oz.	300
Scallops, Bay baked (16-18) 6 oz.	240	**Tuna**, Yellow fin, fresh (4x4x1/4) 6 oz.	240
Oysters 12 avg.	130	**Tuna**, Canned in oil 1/2- 6 oz. can	220
Salmon, Atlantic fresh (3x3x1/4) 5 oz.	258	**Tuna**, Canned in water 1- 6 oz. can	240
Salmon, Smoked ½ lb.	264	**Scallops**, Sea 12 large	240

Eggs, homemade, cooked

Type/Serving Size	Calories	Type/Serving Size	Calories
Eggs 2 medium baked with cheese	265	**Egg** Sandwich 1 regular dry	235
Eggs 3 medium Boiled	225	**Egg** Substitute 2 cups	240

Calories 100-300
Eggs, homemade, cooked

Type/Serving Size	Calories	Type/Serving Size	Calories
Eggs Deviled 4 halves	**290**	**Eggs –** Scrambled 3 medium	**225**
Eggs Fried 2 medium	**210**	**Eggs** Soufflé w/ Cheese 5oz	**275**
Eggs- Poached or boiled 3 medium	**225**		

Beans, homemade, cooked

Type/Serving Size	Calories	Type/Serving Size	Calories
Dry beans, Cooked 1 cup	**240**	**Soybeans** Cooked mature 1 cup	**300**
Refried beans, Regular 1 cup	**280**	**Split peas** Dry, cooked 1 cup	**230**
Refried beans, Fat-free 1 cup	**220**	**Tofu**, Firm 12 oz.	**240**
Soybeans, Dry roasted ½ cup	**260**	**Lentils**, Green/Brown, boiled 8 oz.	**210**
Soybeans Cooked green 1 cup	**260**		

Calories 100-300
Nuts and Seeds

Type/Serving Size	Calories	Type/Serving Size	Calories
Almonds 40	**264**	**Pecans** 40	**245**
Cashews 30	**275**	**Poppy seeds** 6 oz.	**300**
Flax seeds 6 oz.	**265**	**Pumpkin seeds** 6 oz. (6 rounded tbsp.)	**285**
Peanut Butter 3 oz. (6 tbsp.)	**285**	**Sesame seeds** 6 oz.	**300**
Peanuts, Dry roasted 50	**205**	**Sunflower seeds** 5 oz. (5 rounded tbsp.)	**264**
Peanuts, Oil roasted 50	**218**	**Walnuts** ¼ cup	**200**

FRIUTS & JUICES
Juices

Type/Serving Size	Calories	Type/Serving Size	Calories
Apple juice or **cider** 1 pint	**240**	**Lemon juice** 1 pint	**160**
Apricot nectar 1 pint	**280**	**Lime juice** 1 pint	**160**
Cranberry cocktail 1 pint	**290**	**Orange juice** 1 pint	**220**
Cranberry cocktail Reduced-calorie 1 quart	**180**	**Pineapple juice** 1 pint	**280**
Grape juice 1 pint	**300**	**Prune juice** 1 cup	**180**
Grapefruit juice 1 pint	**190**	**Tomato juice** 2 pints	**200**

Calories 100-300
FRIUTS & JUICES
Juices

Type/Serving Size	Calories
Vegetable juice 2 pints	**200**

Fruits

Type/Serving Size	Calories	Type/Serving Size	Calories
Apple 2 large	**200**	**Blackberries** 1 quart	**300**
Applesauce Sweetened 1 cup	**200**	**Blueberries** 1 pint	**160**
Applesauce Unsweetened 1 pint	**200**	**Cantaloupe** 1 quart	**220**
Apricots, Dried 20 halves	**200**	**Cherries,** Sour fresh 1 pint	**160**
Apricots, Fresh 10 medium	**200**	**Cherries,** Sweet fresh 1 pint	**240**
Banana 2 medium	**230**	**Cranberries,** Dried ½ cup	**200**
Cranberries, Fresh 1quart	**200**	**Pear** 2 large	**220**
Fruit cocktail Canned in heavy syrup 1 cup	**180**	**Pineapple** Fresh 1 quart	**300**
Fruit cocktail Canned in light syrup 1 pint	**280**	**Pineapple** Canned in light syrup 1 pint	**260**
Honeydew melon 1 quart	**240**	**Raisins** ½ cup	**250**

Calorie 100-300

Fruits

Type/Serving Size	Calories	Type/Serving Size	Calories
Mandarin oranges 1 pint	200	**Strawberries** 1 quart	200
Papaya 1 medium	120	**Watermelon** 1 quart	200

Vegetables-cooked

Type/Serving Size	Calories	Type/Serving Size	Calories
Artichokes, Cooked 3 medium	180	**Sweet potatoes** or **yams,** baked 1 large -8 oz.	230
Artichoke Hearts Marinated 1 cup	220	**Tomato**, Canned 1 quart	200
Corn, Cooked 1 pint	260	**Tomato**, Dried 1 pint	280
Mixed vegetables, Frozen 1 pint	220	**Potatoes mashed** w milk/ butter 1cup	220
Potato, Baked 1 large - 8 oz.	250		

Calorie 100-300
Dairy products
Milk

Type/Serving Size	Calories	Type/Serving Size	Calories
Milk Whole 1 pint	300	**Buttermilk,** Low-fat 1 pint	220
Milk Reduced-fat 2% 1 pint	240	**Chocolate milk,** Low fat 1 pint	280
Milk Low-fat 1% 1 pint	200	**Rice milk,** Plain 1 pint	240
Milk Fat-free 1 pint	180	**Soy milk,** Plain 1 pint	220

Frozen Desserts

Type/Serving Size	Calories	Type/Serving Size	Calories
Frozen yogurt, 1 cup	240	**Ice cream,** Fat-free 1 cup	180
Frozen yogurt, Fat-free 1 cup	190	**Ice cream,** Fat-free no added sugar 1 pint	280
Ice cream Regular 1 cup	280	**Sherbet** 1 cup	260
Ice cream, Premium ½ cup	260	**Sorbet** Soybean 1 cup	220
Ice cream, Reduced-fat 1 cup	200		

Calories 100-300

Cheese

Type/Serving Size	Calories	Type/Serving Size	Calories
Cheese, Regular (full-fat) 2 oz.	220	**Cream cheese**, Regular 6 tablespoons	300
Cheese, Reduced-fat 3 oz.	240	**Cream cheese** Reduced-fat 6 tablespoons	210
Cheese, fat-free 6 oz.	240	**Ricotta**, Whole milk 1/2 cup	215
Cottage cheese (2%) 1 cup	200	**Ricotta**, Low-fat 1/2 cup	140
Cottage cheese, Fat-free 1 cup	160		

Fats &Oils

Type/Serving Size	Calories	Type/Serving Size	Calories
Bacon fat 2 tablespoons	250	**Oil**, Vegetable 2 tablespoons	240
Butter, Stick whipped 2 tablespoons	240	**Shortening**, Vegetable 2 tablespoons	230
Lard 2 tablespoons	230	**Sour cream**, Regular 1 cup	240
Margarine, Stick 2 tablespoons	200	**Sour cream**, Reduced-fat 1 cup	160
Mayonnaise, Regular 2 tablespoons	200		

Calories 100-300

Breads

Type/Serving Size	Calories	Type/Serving Size	Calories
Bagel, Plain 1 Large (4 oz.)	**300**	**Cornbread** 1 piece (2 oz.)	**190**
Biscuit 1 medium (2 oz.)	**200**	**Croissants** 1 (2 oz.)	**230**
Bread, White 2 slice	**160**	**English muffin** 1 medium	**135**
Bread, Wheat 2 slice	**160**	**Muffin,** Blueberry 1 (2 oz.)	**160**
Bread, Light 4 slice	**160**	**Muffin,** Bran 1 (2 oz.)	**160**
Breadsticks, Soft 2 (2 oz.)	**300**	**Muffin,** Corn 1 (2 oz.)	**175**
Popovers 1 (2 oz.)	**130**	**Roll,** Kaiser 1 medium	**190**
Roll, Hamburger (bun) 1 medium	**125**	**Scone** 1 medium	**150**
Roll, Hot dog (bun) 1 medium	**115**		
Croutons 1 cup	**180**	**Stuffing, bread** 1/2 cup	**195**
French toast 1 slice	**140**	**Stuffing, cornbread** 1/2 cup	**180**
Pancakes 2 (4 inches)	**175**	**Waffle** 1 (2.5 oz.)	**220**

Calories: 100-300

Crackers

Type/Serving Size	Calories	Type/Serving Size	Calories
Animal crackers, Plain 12	170	**Oyster crackers** 40	115
Animal crackers, Icing coated 12	300	**Saltines** 10	120
Graham crackers 4 sheets	220		

Snack Foods

Type/Serving Size	Calories	Type/Serving Size	Calories
Butter Cracker, 10	160	**Popcorn**, Cheese 3 cups	190
Popcorn, Air popped medium bag	240	**Potato chips** Baked 11	120
Popcorn, Microwave medium bag	300	**Potato chips**, Regular 20	150
Popcorn, Microwave, light medium bag	160	**Pretzels**, Large twists 9	110
Popcorn, Oil popped 3 cups	165	**Pretzels**, Small twists 17	110
Popcorn, Caramel 2 cup	300	**Tortilla chips** Regular 13	150

Cereals, Cooked

Type/Serving Size	Calories	Type/Serving Size	Calories
Grits 1 cup	140	**Oatmeal** 1 cup	150

Calories: 100-300

Cereals, Ready to Eat

Type/Serving Size	Calories	Type/Serving Size	Calories
Assorted corn & grain flakes 2¼ cup	300	**Oat cereal,** Toasted 2 cup	220
Granola, Regular 1/2 cup	250	**Raisin Bran** 1 cup	200
Granola, Low-fat 1/2 cup	190		

Rice

Type/Serving Size	Calories	Type/Serving Size	Calories
Rice Brown 1 cup	220	*Rice* Wild 1 cup	170
Rice White 1 cup	260		

Pasta, cooked

Type/Serving Size	Calories	Type/Serving Size	Calories
All flour based pastas 1 cup	210-240	**Spaghetti** 1 cup	200
Egg noodles 1 cup	215	**Quinoa** 1 cup	150
Macaroni 1 cup	200		

Beverages

Beer

Type/Serving Size	Calories	Type/Serving Size	Calories
Beer, Generic 1 can 12 oz.	145	*Coors* Light 1 can 12 oz.	105

Calories 100-300

Beverages
Beer

Type/Serving Size	Calories	Type/Serving Size	Calories
Beer,		**Heileman**	
Light Generic	**100**	Old Style	**145**
1 can 12 oz.		1 can 12 oz.	
Stout,		*Heineken*	
Generic	**120**	1 can 12 oz.	**150**
1 can 12 oz.			
Pale Ale,		*Michelob*	
Generic	**108**	1 can 12 oz.	**160**
1 can 12 oz.			
Anheuser-Busch		*Michelob*	
1 can 12 oz.	**155**	Light	
		1 can 12 oz.	**135**
Anheuser-Busch,		*Miller*	
Light	**110**	Genuine Draft	**150**
1 can 12 oz.		1 can 12 oz.	
Becks	**145**	*Old Milwaukee*	**145**
1 can 12 oz.		1 can 12 oz.	
Budweiser	**145**	*Schlitz*	**145**
1 can 12 oz.		1 can 12 oz.	
Bud Light	**110**	*Stroh's*	**145**
1 can 12 oz.		1 can 12 oz.	
Coors	**140**	*Zima*	**150**
1 can 12 oz.		1 can 12 oz.	

Calories 100-300

Spirits

Type/Serving Size	Calories	Type/Serving Size	Calories
Apricot Brandy		*Highball*	
2 oz.	**160**	8 fl. oz.	**190**
Benedictine		*Margarita*	
2 oz.	**190**	8 fl. oz.	**190**
Bloody Mary		*Martini*	
5 oz.	**120**	2.5 fl. oz.	**155**
Bourbon & Soda		*Rum*	
		100 proof	
5 oz.	**120**	1 jigger	**125**
Brandy,		*Scotch Whiskey*	
100 proof		1 jigger	
1 jigger	**125**		**125**
Brandy,		*Screwdriver*	
94 proof		7.5 fl. oz.	**175**
1 jigger	**115**		
Crème de Cacao		*Sloe Gin*	**125**
2 oz.	**200**	1.5 fl. oz.	
Drambuie		**Southern Comfort**	
1.5 oz.	**165**	1.5 fl. oz.	**180**
Gin & tonic		*Tequila*	
8 fl oz	**195**	1 jigger	**115**
Gin		*Tequila Sunrise*	
100 proof		5 fl. oz.	
1 jigger	**125**		**200**
Tia Maria	**140**	*Whiskey*	
1.5 fl. oz.		100 proof	**125**
		1 jigger	
Vodka		*Whiskey Sour*	
100 proof	**125**	4 fl. oz.	**170**
1 jigger			

Calories 100-300

Wines

Type/Serving Size	Calories	Type/Serving Size	Calories
Burgundy, Red 2 glasses, 8 fl. oz.	**190**	*Madeira* 1 glass, 8 fl. oz.	**160**
Burgundy, White 2 glasses, 8 fl. oz.	**180**	*Marsala* 2 glasses, 8 fl. oz.	**160**
Cabernet Sauvignon 2 glasses, 8 fl. oz.	**180**	*Merlot* 2 glasses, 8 fl. oz.	**160**
Chablis 2 glasses 8 fl. oz.	**170**	*Muscatel* 1 glass, 8 fl. oz.	**160**
Champagne, Dry 1 glass, 4 oz.	**105**	**Port,** Ruby 1 glass, 8 fl. oz.	**160**
Champagne, Pink 1 glass, 4 oz.	**100**	**Port,** White 1 glass, 8 fl. oz.	**170**
Chardonnay 2 glasses, 8 fl. oz.	**180**	*Reisling* 2 glasses, 8 fl. oz.	**180**
Chianti 2 glasses, 8 fl. oz.	**200**	*Rhone* 2 glasses, 8 fl. oz.	**190**
Dubonnet 1 glass, 8 fl. oz.	**160**	*Rose* 2 glasses, 8 fl. oz.	**190**
Liebfraumilch 2 glasses, 8 fl. oz.	**170**	**Sherry,** Dry 1 glass, 8 fl. oz.	**110**
Sangria 1 glass, 8 fl. oz.	**115**	**Vermouth,** Dry 1 glass, 8 fl. oz.	**135**
Sauterne 1 glass, 8 fl. oz.	**115**	*Vermouth*, Sweet 1 glass, 8 fl. oz.	**170**
Sauvignon Blanc 2 glasses, 8 fl. oz.	**160**	**Zinfandel,** Red 2 glasses, 8 fl. oz.	**180**

Calories 100-300

Spirits

Type/Serving Size	Calories	Type/Serving Size	Calories
Sherry,		**Zinfandel,**	
Cream	**160**	White	**160**
2 glasses, 8 fl. oz.		2 glasses, 8 fl. oz.	

Soft Drinks

Type/Serving Size	Calories	*Type/Serving Size*	Calories
7-Up		*Ginger Ale*	
Sweetened	**160**	12 fl. oz.	**140**
12 fl. oz.			
Cherry Cola		*Lemonade*	
Sweetened	**180**	Sweetened	**160**
12 fl. oz.		12 fl. oz.	
Cola		*Lemon-Lime*	
Sweetened	**160**	12 fl. oz.	**140**
12 fl. oz.			
Bitter Lemon	**150**	*Sour Mixer*	**140**
12 fl. oz.		12 fl. oz.	
Collins Mixer	**120**	*Tonic/Quinine*	
12 fl. oz.		12 fl. oz.	**140**
Cream Soda			
Sweetened	**190**		
12 fl. oz.			

Calories 301-500

Assorted fast foods and the 18 food sub-groups

R.L. Erickson C.H.P.

Calories 301-500

Fast foods by Calories

Type/Serving Size	Calories	Type/Serving Size	Calories
Subway Cheese & Egg Breakfast Sandwich 130 g	302	**Kentucky Fried Chicken** Honey BBQ Flavored Sandwich w/ sauce 178 g	310
Papa John's Original Crust Pizza w/ Pepperoni 1/8 of (14" large) 132 g	303	**Kentucky Fried Chicken** Colonels Pies – Apple Pie 1 Slice 113 g	310
Subway Bacon & Egg Breakfast Sandwich 127 g	305	**McDonald's** Chicken McNuggets (6 piece) 108 g	310
Subway Tuna Deli Sandwich 173 g	309	**Pizza Hut** thin'n crispy w/ Meat Lover's (Medium pizza) 1 slice, 116 g	310
Arby's Junior Roast Beef Sandwich 129 g	310	**Pizza Hut** Sicilian Supreme (Medium pizza) 1 slice 134 g	310
Arby's Curly Fries (Small) 99 g	310	**Wendy's** Baked Potato - Plain 284 g	310
Arby's Croissant with Ham 105 g	310	**Wendy's** Jr. Cheeseburger 129 g	310
Burger King Whopper Jr. (w/o Mayo) 147 g	310	**Wendy's** Chili - Large 340 g	310
Burger King Hamburger 121 g	310	**Hardees** Regular Roast Beef 123 g	310
Burger King Hershey's Sundae Pie 79 g	310		

Calories: 301-500

Fast foods by Calories

Type/Serving Size	Calories	Type/Serving Size	Calories
Subway 6" Roasted Chicken Breast Sub 234 g	311	**Subway** Turkey Breast & Bacon (Wrap) 228 g	321
Kentucky Fried Chicken Blazin Strips (3) 129 g	315	**Papa John's** Thin Crust Pizza – The Works (large 14") 1/8, 141 g	322
Burger King Onion Rings - Medium, 91 g	320	**Papa John's** Original Crust Pizza w/ Sausage(14" large) 1/8 142 g	322
Kentucky Fried Chicken Double Choc. Chip Cake 76 g	320	**Burger King** BK Veggie Burger 173 g	330
Burger King Croissan'wich with Egg & Cheese 112 g	320	**Arby's** Jalapeno Bites 111 g	330
Subway Meatball Salad 346 g	320	**Arby's** Biscuit with Ham 125 g	330
Pizza Hut Pan Pizza Supreme (medium) 1 slice, 133 g	320	**McDonald's** Cheeseburger 121 g	330
Pizza Hut Hand Tossed Meat Lover's Pizza (medium) 1 slice, 129 g	320	**Taco Bell** Double Decker Taco 5.75 oz.	330
Taco Bell Nachos 3.5 oz.	320	**Taco Bell** Chili Cheese Burrito 5 oz.	330

Calories: 301-500

Fast foods by Calories

Type/Serving Size	Calories	Type/Serving Size	Calories
Wendy's		**McDonald's**	
Frosty Dairy Dessert - Small 227 g	330	Hot Fudge Sundae 179 g	340
Kentucky Fried Chicken		**Pizza Hut**	
Spicy Crispy Strips (3) 115 g	335	The Big New Yorker w/ Ham 1 slice 168 g	340
Arby's		**Pizza Hut**	
Croissant with Bacon 76 g	340	Pan Pizza Super Supreme (medium pizza) 1 slice 143 g	340
Arby's		**Pizza Hut**	
Arby's Melt w/ Cheddar Sandwich 150 g	340	Sicilian Super Supreme (medium pizza) 1 slice 142 g	340
Arby's		**Taco Bell**	
Hot Ham 'N Swiss Sandwich 170 g	340	Gordita Baja – Chicken or Steak 5.5 oz.	340
Burger King		**Taco Bell**	
Dutch Apple Pie 113 g	340	Chalupa Supreme Chicken— Beef or Steak 5.5 oz.	360
Burger King		**Taco Bell**	
Chicken Tenders – 8 pieces 123 g	340	Chalupa Supreme Chicken— Beef or Steak 5.5 oz.	360
McDonald's		**Papa John's**	
Hotcakes (Plain) 156 g	340	Original Crust Pizza – The Works (large 14") 1/8 160 g	342
McDonald's			
Apple Danish 105 g	340		

Calories 301-500

Fast food

Type/Serving Size	Calories	Type/Serving Size	Calories
		Kentucky Fried Chicken	
Burger King		Hot & Spicy Chicken – Thigh	355
Chicken Whopper Jr. 165 g	350	107 g	
Arby's		**Arby's**	360
Regular Roast Beef Sandwich 157 g	350	Arby's-Q Sandwich 186 g	
Pizza Hut		**Arby's**	360
Sicilian Meat Lover's (Medium pizza) 1 slice 133 g	350	Buttermilk Ranch Dressing (1 pkg) 2 oz.	
Taco Bell		**Arby's**	360
Chalupa Nacho Cheese – Chicken or Steak 5.5 oz.	350	Biscuit with Bacon 96 g	
Taco Bell		**McDonald's**	360
Cheese Quesadilla 4.25 oz.	350	Hot Caramel Sundae 182 g	
Taco Bell		**Pizza Hut**	360
Enchirito- Chicken or Steak or Beef 7.5 oz.	350	Pan Pizza Meat Lover's (medium pizza) 1 slice 133 g	
Wendy's		**Wendy's**	360
Jr. Cheeseburger Deluxe 179 g	350	Blue Cheese Dressing (1pkt) 57 g	
Subway		**Subway**	362
6" BMT Sub 250 g	353	6" Steak & Cheese Sub 253 g	
Subway		**Subway**	362
Steak & Cheese (Wrap) 245 g	353	6" Southwest Chicken 229 g	

Calories 301-500

Fast food

Type/Serving Size	Calories	Type/Serving Size	Calories
Kentucky Fried Chicken		**Taco Bell**	
Popcorn Chicken - Small 99 g	362	Fiesta Burrito – Chicken or Beef 6.5 oz.	370
Arby's		**Wendy's**	
French Toastix (no syrup) 124g	370	Baked Potato – Sour Cream & Chive 312 g	370
Arby's		**Domino's**	
Homestyle Fries (Medium) 142g	370	Classic Hand Tossed – w/ Cheese (12" medium) 2 slices 159 g	375
McDonald's		**Subway**	
Sausage McMuffin 114 g	370	6" Honey Mustard Melt Sub 258 g	376
Taco Bell		**Kentucky Fried Chicken**	
Chalupa Nacho Cheese - Beef 5.5 oz.	370	Honey BBQ Strips (3) 178 g	377
Taco Bell		**Subway**	
Bean Burrito 7 oz.	370	6" Seafood & Crab Sub 252 g	378
Taco Bell		**Kentucky Fried Chicken**	
Enchirito- Beef 7.5 oz.	370	Extra Crispy Chicken - Thigh 118 g	380
Taco Bell		**Burger King**	
Gordita Santa Fe – Chicken Or Steak 5.5 oz.	370	Egg'Wich w/ Canadian Bacon, & Egg 142 g	380
Taco Bell		**McDonald's**	
Fiesta Burrito – Steak-beef 6.5 oz.	370	Fruit 'n Yogurt Parfait 338 g	380

Calories: 301-500

Fast food

Type/Serving Size	Calories	Type/Serving Size	Calories
Pizza Hut The Big New Yorker w/Cheese 1 slice, 174 g	380	**Burger King** French Toast Sticks - 5 Sticks, 112 g	390
Taco Bell Taco Supreme Double Decker 7 oz.	380	**Burger King** Hash Brown Rounds Large 128 g	390
Wendy's Jr. Bacon Cheeseburger 165 g	380	**McDonald's** Cinnamon Roll 95 g	390
Wendy's Taco Salad 468 g	380	**Arby's** Sourdough with Ham 173 g	390
Subway 6" Subway Melt Sub 256 g	384	**Papa John's** Original Crust Pizza w/all the Meats (14" large) 1/8, 160 g	390
Taco Bell Mexican Pizza 6.75 oz.	390	**Subway** 6" Asiago Caesar Chicken Sub 244 g	391
Burger King Whopper Jr 158 g	390	**Papa John's** Thin Crust Pizza w/all the Meats (14" large) 1/8 135 g	393

Calories: 301-500

Fast food

Type/Serving Size	Calories	Type/Serving Size	Calories
Arby's Curly Fries (Medium) 128 g	400	**Pizza Hut** Stuffed Crust w/ Ham (medium pizza) 1 slice 162 g	404
McDonald's Cheese Danish 105 g	400	**Wendy's** Classic Single With Everything 218 g	410
McDonald's Chicken McGrill Sandwich 213 g	400	**Burger King** Egg'Wich w/ Egg & Cheese 140 g	410
Kentucky Fried Chicken Original Recipe Chicken – Breast 153 g	400	**Arby's** Cherry Turnover (Iced) 128 g	410
Subway 12" Veggie Delite Sub 326 g	400	**Kentucky Fried Chicken** Little Bucket Parfait - Lemon Crème 127 g	410
Taco Bell Chalupa Baja-Chicken— Beef or Steak 5.5 oz.	400	**Taco Bell** Burrito Supreme - Chicken 3.75 oz.	410
Taco Bell Taco Salad with Salsa w/o Shell Se16.5 oz.	400	**McDonald's** Sausage Biscuit 112 g	410
Taco Bell Chicken Quesadilla 6 oz.	400	**Wendy's** Spicy Chicken Sandwich 212 g	410
Subway 6" Horseradish Roast Beef Sub 230 g	401	**Hardees** Big Roast Beef Sandwich 165 g	410

Calories: 301-500

Fast food

Type/Serving Size	Calories	Type/Serving Size	Calories
Subway 6" Southwest Steak & Cheese Sub 255 g	412	**Taco Bell** Chalupa Santa Fe - Chicken –beef or Steak 5.5 oz.	420
Subway Asiago Caesar Chicken (Wrap) 244 g	413	**Wendy's** Fries Medium 142 g	420
Subway 6" Cold Cut Trio Sub 254 g	415	**Pizza Hut** Stuffed Crust veggie Lover's (medium pizza) 1 slice 192 g	421
Subway 6" Tuna Sub 252 g	419	**Wendy's** Chicken Breast Fillet Sandwich 207 g	4300
Arby's Apple Turnover (Iced) 128 g	420	**McDonald's** Quarter Pounder 172 g	430
Arby's Sourdough with Bacon 144 g	420	**Pizza Hut** Stuffed Crust Chicken Supreme Pizza (medium) 1 slice, 188 g	432
Burger King Egg'Wich with Canadian bacon, egg, & cheese 155 g	420	**Burger King** Whopper Jr. with cheese 160 g	440
Burger King Chicken Whopper (w/o Mayo) 251 g	420	**Burger King** Cini-minis-4 rolls (Without Vanilla Icing) 108 g	440
Burger King Croissan'wich with Sausage & Cheese 107 g	420	**Burger King** Fresh Baked Cookies 96 g	440

Calories: 301-500

Fast food

Type/Serving Size	Calories	Type/Serving Size	Calories
Arby's		**Kentucky Fried Chicken**	
Croissant with Sausage 102 g	**440**	Original Recipe Sandwich w/sauce 200 g	**450**
Domino's		**Pizza Hut**	
Classic Hand Tossed – Veggie Feast (12" medium) 2 slices, 203.16 g	**440**	The Big New Yorker Veggie Lover's 1 slice, 341 g	**450**
Taco Bell		**Pizza Hut**	
Nachos Supreme 7 oz.	**440**	The Big New Yorker Supreme 1 slice 224 g	**450**
Wendy's		**Domino's**	
Frosty Dairy Dessert Medium 298 g	**440**	Classic Hand Tossed - Hawaiian Feast (12" medium) 2 slices 203.74 g	**451**
Pizza Hut		**McDonald's**	
Stuffed Crust w/ Cheese (medium pizza) 1 slice, 162 g	**445**	Chicken McNuggets (9 piece) 162 g	**460**
Hardee's		**Taco Bell**	
"Hot Dog, with condiments", 160 grams	**450**	Double Burrito Supreme - Chicken or Steak 9 oz.	**460**
Hardee's		**Burger King**	
"Frisco Sandwich, Ham" 187 grams	**450**	Specialty Chicken Sandwich (w/o Mayo) 190 g	**460**
McDonald's		**Arby's**	
French Fries Medium 147 g	**450**	Cheddar Curly Fries 170 g	**460**

Calories: 301-500

Fast food

Type/Serving Size	Calories	Type/Serving Size	Calories
Domino's		**Wendy's**	
Classic Hand Tossed – Deluxe Feast (12" medium) 2 slices 200.8 g	**465**	Baked Potato – Broccoli &Cheese 411 g	**470**
Subway		**Wendy's**	
6" Horseradish Steak & Cheese 254 g	**468**	Chicken Club Sandwich 215 g	**470**
Denny's		**Wendy's**	
Cheesecake Pie (without topping), 4 oz.	**470**	Biggie Fries 159 g	**470**
Arby's		**Kentucky Fried Chicken**	
Vanilla Shake 397 g	**470**	Hot Wing Pieces (6) 135 g	**471**
Arby's		**Hardees**	
Jamocha Shake 397 g	**470**	Chicken Fillet Sandwich 196 g	**480**
Arby's		**Arby's**	
Super Roast Beef Sandwich 245 g	**470**	Chocolate Shake 397 g	**480**
Arby's		**Arby's**	
Mozzerella Sticks 137 g	**470**	Beef 'N Cheddar Sandwich 198 g	**480**
Kentucky Fried Chicken		**Arby's**	
Extra Crispy Chicken – Breast 168 g	**470**	Giant Roast Beef Sandwich 228 g	**480**
McDonald's		**Burger King**	
Filet-O-Fish Sandwich 156 g	**470**	Onion Rings - Large 137 g	**480**

Calories: 301-500

Fast food

Type/Serving Size	Calories	Type/Serving Size	Calories
Burger King		**Burger King**	
BK Homestyle Griller 242 g	**480**	BK 1/4 Lb. Burger 210 g	**490**
McDonald's Bacon, Egg & Cheese Biscuit 152 g	**480**	**Kentucky Fried Chicken** Triple Crunch Sandwich w/ sauce 189 g	**490**
Pizza Hut Catavini Pasta 357 g	**480**	**Kentucky Fried Chicken** Colonels Pies – Pecan Pie Slice 113 g	**490**
Pizza Hut Stuffed Crust Supreme (medium pizza) 1 slice 196 g	**487**	**McDonald's** Crispy Chicken Sandwich Serving Size: 219 g	**500**
Pizza Hut Spaghetti w/ Marinara 473 g	**490**	**Arby's** Cool Ranch Baked Potato, 12.3 oz.	**500**
McDonald's Sausage Biscuit with Egg 162 g	**490**	**Arby's** Baked Potato w/Butter & Sour Cream 320 g	**500**

Calories: 301-500

Meat—Alphabetically

Beef, cooked

Type/Serving Size	Calories	Type/Serving Size	Calories
Chuck roast, Arm 8 oz.	**492**	**Pot roast,** Round 6 oz.	**486**
Flank steak 8 oz.	**466**	**Prime rib** ¼ lb.	**485**
Ground beef, Regular 6 oz.	**489**	**Sirloin steak** 8 oz.	**452**
Ground beef, Lean 6 oz.	**429**	**Tenderloin** 8 oz.	**480**
T-bone or Porterhouse steak ¼ lb.	**340**	**Ground beef**, Extra lean 6 oz.	**380**

Lamb, cooked

Type/Serving Size	Calories	Type/Serving Size	Calories
Lamb chops 8 oz.	**492**	**Lamb leg** 6 oz.	**440**

Pork-cooked

Type/Serving Size	Calories	Type/Serving Size	Calories
Ground Pork ¼ lb.	**339**	**Sausage,** Italian ¼ lb.	**430**
Ham 8 oz.	**359**	**Sausage,** Polish ¼ lb.	**450**
Pork chops 8 oz.	**479**	**Sausage,** Smoked ¼ lb.	**380**
Pork tenderloin 8 oz.			**372**

Poultry

Chicken, cooked Homestyle

Type/Serving Size	Calories	Type/Serving Size	Calories
Breast, Skin 8 oz.	452	**Thighs,** No skin 8 oz.	440
Breast, No skin 8 oz.	372	**Wings**, Roasted 5	500
Breast, Deli cut 8 oz.	360	**Drumstick** Roasted w/skin 8 oz.	452
Thighs, Skin 6 oz.	420	**Whole chicken** Roasted w/skin 8 oz.	370

Turkey, cooked homestyle

Type/Serving Size	Calories	Type/Serving Size	Calories
Turkey Breast, Deli 8 oz.	340	**Turkey**, Light meat, no skin 8 oz.	320
Turkey, Dark meat, skin 8 oz.	492	**Ground turkey,** Lean 8 oz.	452
Turkey, Dark meat, No skin 8 oz.	426	**Ground turkey** Extra-lean 8 oz.	320
Turkey, Light meat, skin 8 oz.	372		

Calories: 301-500—alphabetically

Fish & seafood cooked

Type/Serving Size	Calories	Type/Serving Size	Calories
Catfish ½ lb.	326	**Orange Roughy** 1 lb.	400
Cod 1 lb.	480	**Salmon**, Atlantic fresh ½ lb.	412
Crab, Blue fresh 1 lb.	480	**Salmon,** Smoked 12 oz.	400
Crab, Blue canned 3 cups	420	**Scallops,** Bay 12 oz.	480
Crab, Imitation 1 lb.	480	**Sea Scallops**, 18 large	360
Halibut, Atlantic ½ lb.	320	**Tuna**, Yellowfin, fresh 12 oz.	480
Lobster 12 oz.	440	**Tuna,** Canned in oil 1 cup	440
Mussels 10 oz.	484	**Tuna,** Canned in water 2 cup	480

Eggs, cooked

Type/Serving Size	Calories	Type/Serving Size	Calories
Eggs Benedict 1 serving	410	**Deviled Eggs** 6 halves	435
Eggs, curried 6 oz.	372	**Eggs, fried** 3	315
Eggs w/low fat cheese sauce 6 oz.	360	**3-egg omelet, no cheese** 4 oz.	440
Eggs w/cheese sauce 6 oz.	420	**Soufflé w/cheese** 8 oz.	440

Calories: 301-500 – alphabetically

Beans and peas, cooked
(See chart 100-300)

Calories: 301-500 — alphabetically

Nuts

Type/Serving Size	Calories	Type/Serving Size	Calories
Almonds	330	**Poppy seeds**	400
50		½ cup	
Cashews	330	**Pumpkin seeds**	380
36		½ cup	
Flax seeds	380	**Sesame seeds**	400
8 oz.		½ cup	
Peanut Butter		**Sunflower seeds**	410
4 tablespoons	380	½ cup	
Peanuts, dry roasted		**Walnuts**	400
100	410	½ cup	
Pecans			
75	460		

Fruits juices

Type/Serving Size	Calories	Type/Serving Size	Calories
Apple juice or cider	480	**Prune juice**	360
1 quart		1 pint	
Grapefruit juice	380	**Tomato juice**	400
1 quart		½ gallon	
Orange juice	440	**Vegetable juice**	400
1 quart		½ gallon	

221

Calories: 301-500— alphabetically
Whole Fruits and Vegetables
See 100-300 Cal charts

Calories: 301-500— alphabetically

Dairy products

Milk
See 101-300 Cal charts

Yogurt

Type/Serving Size	Calories	Type/Serving Size	Calories
Whole milk,		**Fat-free,**	
plain	**360**	plain	
1 pint		1 quart	**400**
Low-fat,		**Low-fat,**	
plain	**440**	flavored	
1 quart		1 pint	**460**
Frozen yogurt,		**Frozen yogurt,**	
regular	**480**	Fat-free	**380**
2 cups		2 cups	

Cheese

Type/Serving Size	Calories	Type/Serving Size	Calories
Cheese,		**Cottage cheese,**	
(Full-fat) regular	**440**	Fat-free	**320**
4 oz.		2 cups	
Cheese,		**Cream cheese,**	
Reduced-fat	**360**	Regular	**400**
4 oz.		8 tablespoons	
Cheese,		**Cream cheese,**	
Fat-free	**360**	Reduced-fat	**350**
8 oz.		10 tablespoons	
Cottage cheese		**Cream cheese,**	
(2%)	**400**	Fat-free	**360**
2 cups		12 oz.	
Feta cheese		**Ricotta,**	**420**
4 oz.	**320**	Low-fat	
		1½ cups	

<u>Calories: 301-500— alphabetically</u>
<u>Dairy products</u>

<u>Cheese</u>

<u>Type/Serving Size</u>	Calories	<u>Type/Serving Size</u>	Calories
Mozzarella part-Skim cheese 4 oz.	320	String cheese 6 oz.	420
Ricotta, Whole milk 1 cup	430		

<u>Frozen Desserts</u>

<u>Type/Serving Size</u>	Calories	<u>Type/Serving Size</u>	Calories
Ice cream, Regular 1½ cups	420	**Ice cream,** Fat-free w/ no added sugar 2 cups	320
Ice cream, Premium 12 oz.	390	**Sherbet** 1½ cups	390
Ice cream, Reduced-fat 2 cups	400	**Sorbet** 2 cups	440
Ice cream, Fat-free 2 cups	360		

<u>Fats & oils</u>

<u>Type/Serving Size</u>	Calories	<u>Type/Serving Size</u>	Calories
Bacon fat 4 tablespoons	500	**Mayonnaise**, Low-fat 6 oz.	420
Butter, stick 4 oz., 1stick	400	**Mayonnaise,** Fat-free 16 oz.	320
Butter, whipped 3 oz.	450	**Oil**, Vegetable 4 tablespoons	480

223

Calories: 301-500—alphabetically

Oils and Fats

Type/Serving Size	Calories	Type/Serving Size	Calories
Lard 2 oz.	460	**Shortening,** Vegetable 4 tablespoons	460
Margarine, stick 4 tablespoons	400	**Sour cream,** Regular 6 oz.	360
Mayonnaise, Regular 4 tablespoons	400	**Sour cream,** Reduced-fat 8 oz.	320

Sweets

Type/Serving Size	Calories	Type/Serving Size	Calories
Chocolate syrup 4 oz.	400	**Pancake syrup,** Regular 4 oz.	440
Honey 4 oz.	420	**Pancake syrup,** Reduced-calorie 8 oz.	400
Jam/jelly 4 oz.	400	**Sugar,** White or brown 4 oz.	360
Maple syrup 4 oz.	400	**Sugar,** White or brown 4 oz.	360

Breads

Type/Serving Size	Calories	Type/Serving Size	Calories
Biscuit, Homemade 2 medium (2 oz.)	400	**Muffin,** Corn 2 (2 oz.)	325
Bread, White 4 slices	320	**Popovers** 3 (2 oz.)	390
Bread, Wheat 4 slices	320	**Dinner Roll,** 4 medium	340

Calories: 301-500—alphabetically

Breads

Type/Serving Size	Calories	Type/Serving Size	Calories
Breadsticks, Soft 3 (2 oz.)	**450**	**Roll**, Hamburger 4 medium	**500**
Cornbread 2 piece (2 oz.)	**380**	**Roll,** Hot dog 3 medium	**345**
Croissants 2 (2 oz.)	**460**		**500**
Muffin, Blueberry 2 (2 oz.)	**320**	**Roll,** Kaiser 2 medium	**380**
Muffin, Bran 2 (2 oz.)	**320**	**Scone** 3 medium	**350**

Bread Products

Type/Serving Size	Calories	Type/Serving Size	Calories
Croutons 2 cups	**360**	**Stuffing, bread** 1 cup	**390**
French toast 3 slices	**420**	**Stuffing, cornbread** 1 cup	**360**
Pancakes 4 (4 inches)	**350**	**Waffle** 2 (2.5 oz.)	**440**
Pretzel, soft 1 large	**340**		**360**

Snack Foods

Type/Serving Size	Calories	Type/Serving Size	Calories
Popcorn, Oil popped 6 cups	**330**	**Potato chips**, Regular 60	**450**
Popcorn, Caramel 3 cups	**450**	**Pretzels,** Large twists 27	**330**
Popcorn, Cheese 6 cups	**380**	**Pretzels**, Small twists 51	**330**
Potato chips, Baked 44	**500**	**Tortilla chips**, Baked Regular rounds, 40	**470**

Calories: 301-500 - alphabetically

Cereals, cooked

Type/Serving Size	Calories	Type/Serving Size	Calories
Grits, 3 cups	**420**	**Oatmeal**, 3 cups	**450**

Cereals, Ready to Eat

Type/Serving Size	Calories	Type/Serving Size	Calories
Granola, Regular 1 cup	**500**	**Assorted corn & grain flakes** 3 cups	**400**
Granola, Low-fat 1 cup	**380**	**Raisin Bran** 2 cups	**400**
Oat cereal, Toasted 3 cups	**330**		**330**

Crackers

Type/Serving Size	Calories	Type/Serving Size	Calories
Animal crackers, plain 30	**425**	**Saltines** 30	**360**
Animal crackers, iced 18	**450**	**Butter Crackers**, 20	**320**

Rice, cooked

Type/Serving Size	Calories	Type/Serving Size	Calories
Rice, brown 2 cup	**440**	**Rice, wild** 2 cup	**340**
Rice, white 1 ½ cups	**390**	**Quinoa**, 1½ cups	**450**

Pasta–cooked

Type/Serving Size	Calories	Type/Serving Size	Calories
All flour based pastas 2 cups	**410-440**	**Macaroni** 2 cups	**400**
Egg noodles 2 cups	**430**	**Spaghetti** 2 cups	**400**

Calories: 501-699

Assorted fast foods and the 18 food sub-groups

R.L. Erickson C.H.P.

Calories: 501-699

Fast foods by Calories

Type/Serving Size	Calories	Type/Serving Size	Calories
Subway 6" Meatball Sub 284 g	501	**Taco Bell** Double Burrito Supreme Beef 10.25 oz.	510
Pizza Hut Stuffed Crust Super Supreme (medium pizza) 1 slice, 198 g	505	**Denny's** Country fried potatoes 6 oz.	515
Kentucky Fried Chicken Hot & Spicy Chicken Breast 180 g	505	**Domino's** Classic Hand Tossed w/ Cheese (14" large) 2 slices 219 g	516
Domino's Classic Hand TossedBarbeque Feast (12" medium) 2 slices, 192 g	507	**Denny's** Buffalo Chicken Salad 16 oz.	516
Domino's Classic Hand TossedAmerica's Favorite Feast (12" medium) 2 slices, 204.82 g	508	**Denny's** Grilled chicken sandwich 11 oz.	520
Subway 12" Turkey Breast Sub 440 g	508	**Dairy Queen** Blizzards Choc. or Butterfinger 12 oz.	520
Dairy Queen Dipped cone reg. 8.3 oz.	510	**Arby's** Sourdough with Sausage 170 g	520
Dairy Queen Banana split 13 oz.	510	**Arby's** Roast Chicken Club Sandwich 278 g	520

Calories: 301-500

Fast foods by calories

Type/Serving Size	Calories	Type/Serving Size	Calories
Taco Bell		**Subway**	
7 - Layer Burrito 10 oz.	520	12" Roast Beef Sub 440 g	528
Subway		**Arby's**	
12" Ham Sub 438 g	522	Hot Ham 'N Swiss Sub 278 g	530
Pizza Hut		**McDonald's**	
Stuffed Crust Pepperoni Lover's (medium pizza) 1 slice 192 g	525	Quarter Pounder with Cheese 200 g	530
Subway		**Denny's**	
6" Caesar Italian BMT 254 g	530	Potato pancakes 13 oz.	530
Wendy's **Baked Potato** –		**Denny's**	
Bacon & Cheese 380 g	530	Ham & Swiss on rye 9 oz.	533
Hardees	530	**Denny's**	
Fisherman's Fillet 221 g		Seniors menu triple play 8 oz.	537
Subway		**Arby's** Baked Potato	540
12" Turkey Breast & Ham Sub 458 g	534	Broccoli 'N Cheddar 384 g	
Domino's		**Burger King**	
Classic Hand Tossed - Pepperoni Feast (12" medium) 2 slices, 196.08 g	535	Double Cheeseburger 189 g	540
Arby's	540	**McDonald's**	
Chicken Breast Fillet Sandwich 208 g		French Fries Large 176 g	540

Calories: 301-500

Fast foods by calories

Type/Serving Size	Calories	Type/Serving Size	Calories
McDonald's		**Denny's**	
Big N' Tasty Sandwich 251 g	540	Banana royale 10 oz.	548
Dairy Queen		**Burger King**	
Cheeseburger Deluxe double 8.5 oz.	540	King Supreme Sandwich 196 g	550
Pizza Hut		**Burger King**	
Stuffed Crust Meat Lover's (medium pizza) 1 slice, 196 g	543	Onion Rings - King Size, 159 g	550
McDonald's		**Subway**	
Ham, Egg & Cheese Bagel 218 g	550	12" Honey Mustard Turkey w/ Cucumber 464 g	550
Domino's		**Pizza Hut**	
Classic Hand Tossed – Bacon Cheeseburger Feast (12" medium) 2 slices, 198.38 g	550	Ham & Cheese Sandwich 276 g	550
Kentucky Fried Chicken		**Kentucky Fried Chicken**	
Triple Crunch Zinger Sandwich w/ sauce 210 g	550	Honey BBQ Crunch Melt 231 g	556

R.L. Erickson C.H.P.

Calories: 501-699

Fast foods by calories

Type/Serving Size	Calories	Type/Serving Size	Calories
Denny's Fried shrimp dinner 8 oz.	**558**	**McDonald's** Strawberry Shake 444 ml	**560**
Denny's Grilled Alaskan Salmon Dinner 8 oz.	**558**	**Arby's** Homestyle Fries Large, 213 g	**560**
Burger King Vanilla Shake - Small 305 g	**560**	**Pizza Hut** Supreme Pasta 396 g	**560**
Burger King Specialty Chicken Sandwich 204 g	**560**	**Denny's** Ultimate Omelette 13 oz.	**564**
Domino's Classic Hand Tossed - MeatZZa Feast (12" medium) 2 slices, 216.24 g	**560**	**Wendy's** Great Biggie Fries 190 g	**570**
McDonald's Strawberry Shake 444 ml	**560**	**Hardee's** Famous Star 245 g	**570**
Dairy Queen Chocolate Shake- small, 14 oz.	**560**	**Arby's** Chicken Finger Salad (Fresh) 367 g	**570**
Dairy Queen Heath Blizzard small, 12 oz.	**560**	**McDonald's** Vanilla Shake 444 ml	**570**

Calories: 501-699

Fast foods by calories

Type/Serving Size	Calories	Type/Serving Size	Calories
McDonald's		**Arby's**	
Oreo® McFlurry	570	Chicken Finger Snack	580
337 g		181 g	
Domino's			
Classic Hand Tossed -		**Burger King**	
ExtravaganZZa Feast		Chicken Whopper	
(12" medium)	576	272 g	580
2 slices 244.94 g			
Burger King		**Subway**	
Bacon Double Cheeseburger	580	12" Subway Club Sub	588
193 g		506 g	
McDonald's		**McDonald's**	
Chocolate Shake		Big Mac	590
444 ml	580	216 g	
Pizza Hut		**McDonald's**	
Personal Pan Pizza w/ Ham	580	Big N' Tasty	
1 pizza, 260 g		With Cheese Sandwich	590
		265 g	
Wendy's		Dairy Queen	
Big Bacon Classic	580	Peanut Butter Cup	
282 g		Blizzard	590
		small, 12 oz.	
Pizza Hut		**Arby's**	
Spaghetti w/ Meat Sauce	600	Chicken Bacon 'N Swiss	
467 g		Sandwich	610
		213 g	
McDonald's		**McDonald's**	
Hotcakes		Butterfinger McFlurry	
(Margarine, 2 pats & Syrup)	600	348 g	620
228 g			
Burger King		**Kentucky Fried**	
French Fries		**Chicken**	
King Size (salted)	600	Popcorn Chicken	620
194 g		Large, 170 g	

Calories: 501-699

Fast foods by calories

Type/Serving Size	Calories	Type/Serving Size	Calories
Burger King Whopper (w/o Mayo) 283 g	**600**	**Burger King** Chocolate Shake (Syrup added) Small 333 g	**620**
Denny's Key Lime Pie 6 oz.	**600**	**Burger King** Strawberry Shake (Syrup added) Small 333 g	**620**
Domino's Classic Hand Tossed – Veggie Feast (14" large) 2 slices, 278.12 g	**605**	**Arby's** Curly Fries Large, 198 g	**620**
Kentucky Fried Chicken Honey BBQ 6 Pieces, 189 g	**607**	**Subway** 12" Roasted Chicken Breast Sub 468 g	**622**
Hardees Monster Roast Beef 208 g	**610**	**Domino's** Classic Hand TossedHawaiian Feast (14" large) 2 slices, 282.96 g	**623**
McDonald's French Fries Super Size 198 g	**610**	**Denny's** Chicken Strips Dinner, 10 oz.,	**635**
Domino's Classic Hand Tossed Deluxe Feast (14" large) 2 slices, 272.56 g	**628**	**Pizza Hut** Supreme Sandwich 292 g	**640**
Pizza Hut Personal Pan Pizza w/cheese 1 pizza, 263 g	**630**	**Arby's** Chicken Finger 4-Pack 192 g	**640**
McDonald's M&M McFlurry 348 g	**630**		

Calories: 501-699

Fast foods by calories

Type/Serving Size	Calories
McDonald's Nestles Crunch McFlurry 348 g	630
Arby's Turkey Sub 306 g	630
Arby's Big Montana Sandwich 313 g	630
Denny's Cherry Pie 7 oz.	630
Denny's Bacon, Lettuce and Tomato Sandwich 6 oz.	634
Denny's Eggs Benedict 15 oz.	695
Hardees Bacon Swiss Crispy Chicken Sandwich 217 g	670
Dairy Queen Home style Ultimate Burger 9.5 oz.	670
Denny's Classic Burger 11 oz.	673

Type/Serving Size	Calories
Dairy Queen Choc. Sandwich Cookie Blizzard regular, 16 oz.	640
Denny's T-bone Steak Dinner 12 oz.	642
Arby's Deluxe Baked Potato 361 g	650
Hardee's All Star Burger 266 g	660
Denny's Garden Burger 11 oz.	665
Taco Bell Grilled Stuft Burrito Steak 10.4 oz.	690
McDonald's Spanish Omelet Bagel 258 g	690
Domino's Classic Hand Tossed - Barbeque Feast (14" large) 2 slices, 262.16 g	692
Domino's Classic Hand Tossed - America's Favorite Feast (14" large) 2 slices 282.96 g	698

Calories: 501-699

Fast foods by calories

Beef, cooked

Type/Serving Size	Calories	Type/Serving Size	Calories
Brisket, Lean & fat, Braised 6 oz.	670	**Steak**, Porterhouse, lean & fat 8 oz.	680
Chuck, Pot roast, lean & fat 6 oz.	600	**Steak**, T-bone, lean & fat, broiled 8 oz.	700
Chuck, Stewing meat, lean & fat 6 oz.	560	**Tenderloin**, Lean & fat, broiled 8 oz.	613
Rib roasted, Lean & fat 6 oz.	667	**Top Loin**, Lean & fat, broiled 8 oz.	667
Rib Eye, Lean & fat, broiled 8 oz.	657	**Hamburger**, Lean & fat, broiled 8 oz.	640
Round, Eye of, Lean & fat, roasted 8 oz.	547	**Corned Beef** 8 oz.	630
Rump Roast, Lean & fat 6 oz.	570	**Beef Liver**, Fried 9 oz.	600
Sirloin, Lean & fat, broiled 8 oz.	640	**Veal Cutlet**, Lean & fat broiled 10 oz.	600
		Veal Rib Roast 8 oz.	613

Calories: 501-699

Lamb, cooked

Type/Serving Size	Calories	Type/Serving Size	Calories
Lamb Chop, Arm, braised lean & fat 6 oz.	600	**Lamb Leg**, Lean & fat, roasted 8 oz.	640
Lamb Chop, Loin, lean & fat, broiled 8 oz.	667	**Lamb Shoulder**, Lean & fat, roasted 6 oz.	580
Lamb Chop, Rib, lean & fat, broiled 6 oz.	699		

Pork, cooked

Type/Serving Size	Calories	Type/Serving Size	Calories
Center Loin Chop, Broiled/grilled 12 oz.	660	**Tenderloin,** Roasted 12 oz.	600
Loin Chop, Broiled/grilled 12 oz.	699	**Ham,** Lean and fat 8 oz.	667
Rib Chops 10 oz.	616	**Pork Sausages**, Broiled/grilled 8 oz.	640

Calories: 501-699

Poultry, fried or baked

Type/Serving Size	Calories	Type/Serving Size	Calories
Chicken breast, Meat and skin w/batter 8 oz.	588	**Chicken,** Whole, roasted, meat and skin 12 oz.	555
Chicken drumstick, Meat and skin, 8 oz.	628	**Chicken Breast Patties** 7 oz.	500
Chicken leg, Meat and skin, w/batter 8 oz.	640		

Poultry, fried or baked

Turkey

Type/Serving Size	Calories	Type/Serving Size	Calories
Turkey, Light meat and skin roasted 10 oz.	642	**Turkey,** Meat only, roasted 12 oz.	651

Fish and seafood, grilled or baked

Type/Serving Size	Calories	Type/Serving Size	Calories
Catfish 16 oz.	692	**Salmon**, Atlantic, fresh 12 oz.	619
Cod 20 oz.	600	**Salmon,** Smoked 20 oz.	608
Crab, Blue, fresh 20 oz.	600	**Scallops,** Bay 16 oz.	640
Crab, Blue, canned 5 cups	699	**Scallops**, Sea 30 large	600

Calories: 501-699

Fish and Seafood-grilled or baked

Type/Serving Size	Calories	Type/Serving Size	Calories
Crab, Imitation 20 oz.	**600**	**Tuna,** Yellowfin, fresh 16 oz.	**640**
Halibut, Atlantic 16 oz.	**640**	**Tuna,** Canned in oil 1½ cups	**660**
Lobster 16 oz.	**586**	**Tuna,** Canned in water 2½ cups	**600**
Mussels 12 oz.	**600**		

Eggs

Type/Serving Size	Calories	Type/Serving Size	Calories
Eggs with cheese sauce 10 oz.	**699**	**Eggs Curried** 10 oz.	**610**
Eggs a la King 5 oz.	**690**	**Eggs Florentine** 2	**520**
Eggs Antoine 5 oz.	**590**	**Eggs Romano** 2	**630**

Beans, cooked

Type/Serving Size	Calories	Type/Serving Size	Calories
Dry beans 2½ cups	**600**	**Soybeans** Dry roasted 1 cup	**540**
Refried beans, Regular 2½ cup	**699**	**Soybeans** Cooked mature 2 cups	**600**
Refried beans, Fat-free 3 cups	**660**	**Split peas** (dry), Cooked, 3 cups	**690**

Calories: 501-699

Nuts and Seeds
See 301-500 calorie chart

Fats and Oils
See 301-500 calorie chart

Fruits
See 301-500 calorie chart

Vegetables
See 301-500 calorie chart

Calories: 501-699 - alphabetically

Dairy Products

Milk

Type/Serving Size	Calories	Type/Serving Size	Calories
Whole milk 1 quart	**600**	**Chocolate milk, fat-free** 1 quart	580

Yogurt

Type/Serving Size	Calories	Type/Serving Size	Calories
Whole milk, Plain, 3 cups	**540**	**Frozen yogurt**, Regular 2½ cup	**600**
Low-fat, Flavored, 3 cups	**690**		

Calories: 501-699-Alphabetically
Dairy products

Cheese

Type/Serving Size	Calories	Type/Serving Size	Calories
Cheese Full-fat regular 6 oz.	**660**	**Cottage cheese**, fat-free 4 cups	**640**
Cheese, Reduced-fat 8 oz.	**640**	**Ricotta,** Whole milk 1½ cups	**645**
Cottage 2% cheese 3 cups	**600**	**Ricotta,** Low-fat 2 cups	**560**

Frozen Desserts

Type/Serving Size	Calories	Type/Serving Size	Calories
Ice cream, Regular 2 cups	**560**	**Ice cream**, Fat-free no added sugar 5 cups	**699**
Ice cream, Premium 1 cup	**520**	**Sherbet** 2½ cups	**650**
Ice cream, Reduced-fat 3 cups	**600**	**Sorbet** 2½ cups	**550**
Ice cream, Fat-free 3 cups	**540**		

Breads
See 301-500 calorie chart

Sweets
See 301-500 calorie chart

Cereals
See 301-500 calorie chart

<u>Calories: 501-699 – alphabetically</u>

<u>Rice, cooked</u>

<u>Type/Serving Size</u>	Calories	<u>Type/Serving Size</u>	Calories
<u>Rice, Brown</u> 3 cups	540	<u>Rice Wild</u> 4 cups	680
<u>Rice, White</u> 2 cups	520		

<u>Pasta, cooked</u>

<u>Type/Serving Size</u>	Calories	<u>Type/Serving Size</u>	Calories
<u>All flour pastas</u> 3 cups	630- 699	<u>Macaroni,</u> 3 cups	600
<u>Egg noodles</u>, 3 cups	645	<u>Spaghetti,</u> 3 cups	600

<u>Beverages</u>
See 100-300 calorie chart

Cautionary Foods

As a consumer, food is viewed as any other commodity, and you want the most for your money. The food industry, understanding this, provides low cost high calorie products, engineered to have the right taste, smell, and texture to appeal to both your cravings and sense of savings.

Individual foods that contain more than 700 calories should be viewed as *cautionary*. Once an individual food exceeds 700 calories, it becomes a percentage drain on your daily calorie maximum.

If, for example, your second-day daily calorie maximum was 1500 calories, and you consumed an 850-calorie burger, over 50% of your daily calories would be used on one food.

There is nothing wrong in eating high calorie foods; however, it is recommended that these foods be eaten in portions over time and not in one sitting. Using the example, above you could eat this 850-calorie burger in quarters over the course of the day. You enjoy the food more often and stay within the calorie range.

Remember, in order to burn excess stored body fat, it is essential to stay within your daily calorie maximums and start to think of food as energy (calories) first and view taste, smell, and texture as secondary.

The following are examples of some high calorie individual foods on the market. These are random examples.

Calories: 700+ - Cautionary foods

Fast food

Type/Serving Size	Calories	Type/Serving Size	Calories
Arby's Philly Beef 'N Swiss Sub 311 g	700	**Subway** 12" Southwest Chicken 458 g	724
McDonald's Steak, Egg & Cheese Bagel 245 g	700	**Arby's** Roast Ham & Swiss Sandwich (Fresh) 360 g	730
Burger King BK Big Fish Sandwich 262 g	710	**Taco Bell** Grilled Stuft Burrito - Beef 10.3 oz.	730
Dairy Queen Peanut Buster Parfait Regular	720	**Domino's** Classic Hand Tossed - Pepperoni Feast (14" large) 2 slices, 270.26 g	732
Hardee's Frisco Burger, 219 g	720	**Pizza Hut** Personal Pan Pizza w/ one added meat topping 1 pizza, 291 g	740
Kentucky Fried Chicken Blazin Twister 246 g	719	**Kentucky Fried Chicken** Crispy Honey Twister 270 g	744
Burger King Vanilla Shake - Medium 397 g	720	**Dairy Queen** Butterfinger Blizzard regular	750
Burger King BK Smokehouse Cheddar Griller 241 g	720	**Subway** 12" Honey Mustard Melt Sub 516 g	752
Subway 12" Steak & Cheese Sub 506 g	724	**Domino's** Classic Hand Tossed - MeatZZa Feast (14" large) 2 slices, 292.78 g	753
Subway 12" Seafood & Crab Sub 504 g	756	**Domino's** Classic Hand Tossed - ExtravaganZZa Feast (14" large) 2 slices, 329.46 g	774

Calories: 700+ - Cautionary foods

Fast food

Type/Serving Size	Calories	Type/Serving Size	Calories
Arby's Roast Beef Sub 334 g	760	**Arby's** Italian Sub 312 g	780
Arby's Roast Turkey & Swiss Sandwich (Fresh) 360 g	760	**Burger King** Strawberry Shake (Syrup added) Medium, 425 g	780
Burger King Whopper 304 g	760	**Subway** 12" Asiago Caesar Chicken Sub 488 g	782
Taco Bell Nachos Bell Grande 11 oz.	760	**Burger King** Chocolate Shake (Syrup added) Medium 425 g	790
Domino's Classic Hand Tossed Bacon Cheeseburger Feast (14" large) 2 slices 274.92 g	763	**Hardee's** Super star 324 g	790
Subway 12" Subway Melt Sub 512 g	768	**Subway** 12" Horseradish Roast Beef Sub 460 g	802
Dairy Queen Chocolate Shake Regular	770	**Arby's** Roast Beef & Swiss Sandwich (Fresh) 360 g	810
Kentucky Fried Chicken Chunky Chicken Pot Pie 368 g	770	**Denny's** Chili Cheese Fries	816
Dairy Queen Heath Blizzard Large	820	**Denny's** Garlic Mushroom Swiss Burger	872
Arby's Roast Chicken Caesar Sandwich (Fresh) 363 g	820	**Denny's** Bacon Cheddar Burger	875

Calories: 700 + - Cautionary foods

Fast food

Type/Serving Size	Calories	Type/Serving Size	Calories
Subway 12" Southwest Steak & Cheese Sub 510 g	**824**	**Burger King** Double Whopper (w/o Mayo) 380 g	**900**
Subway 12" Cold Cut Trio Sub 508 g	**830**	**Subway** 12" BMT Sub 500 g	**906**
Denny's Classic Burger with Cheese	**836**	**Denny's** Big Texas BBQ Burger	**929**
Subway 12" Tuna Sub 304 g	**838**	**Subway** 12"Horseradish Steak & Cheese 508 g	**936**
Burger King Whopper With Cheese 329 g	**850**	**Denny's** Buffalo Wings 12 pc.	**940**
Pizza Hut Spaghetti w/ Meatballs 537 g	**850**	**Dairy Queen** Chocolate. Chip Cookie Dough Blizzard Large	**950**
Taco Bell Taco Salad with Salsa 19 oz.	**850**	**Burger King** Double Whopper With Cheese (w/o Mayo) 405 g	**990**
Subway 12"Meatball Sub 568 g	**1,002**	**Taco Bell** Mucho Grande Nachos 18 oz.	**1,320**
Hardee's Monster Burger 288 g	**1,060**	**Schlotzsky's** Chicken Club Large, 31 oz.	**1,352**
Burger King Double Whopper W/ Cheese 426 g	**1,150**	**Schlotzsky's** Turkey Original Large 39.4oz	**2,083**
Denny's Double Decker Burger	**1,247**		
Schlotzsky's Western Vegetarian Large -23.1oz	**1,261**		

Mix and match menus

The System provides you with a new approach to calories. By having foods broken into 100- and 200-calorie sections, you can compare foods that have the same energy potential. Mixing and matching can now be enjoyable and interesting.

The System's top *base number* average weekly calorie amount (for certain individuals over 380 pounds) is 3,582 Calories. Even at this higher calorie amount, it is not recommended to eat groups of single foods exceeding 700 calories. *Remember, a healthy digestive tract uses approximately 10% of the calories you consume each day in digesting the very foods you eat.*

It is essential, therefore, to keep the digestive tract active by consuming smaller portions, but during more meals (5-7 including snacks). If we divided the national per-capita average calorie intake, 3,400 by 5, we would get about 680 calories.

This would be less than a MacDonald's steak, egg, and cheese bagel (700 Calories), a Dairy Queen Peanut Buster Parfait (720 Calories), or a Burger King BK Big fish sandwich (710 Calories).

Imagine how foods like a Burger King Double Whopper with cheese (1150 Calories), a Denny's Double Decker Burger (1247 Calories) or Schlotzsky's Turkey Original Large (2083 Calories) would affect a 1500, 2500 or even 3500 weekly calorie average. As stated earlier, this is not to say these foods cannot be eaten. They just need to be eaten over time and not in one sitting.

The following are examples of menus and how matching the calorie contents and mixing different foods can be easy and interesting.

A *meal* refers to any food consumed during the day (24-hour period) and includes snacks, drinks containing calories, candy breaks, etc.

Breakfast

0-600 Calorie Meals

Breakfast

0-600 Calorie meals

Type of food	Cal	Type of food	Cal
Apple 1 medium	80	**Tea** No sweetener	1

Total calories 81

Type of food	Cal	Type of food	Cal	Type of food	Cal
Corn grits* Plain instant, 1 packet	80	**Peach** 1 medium	40	**Sparkling water** 12 oz.	0

Total calories 120

Type of food	Cal	Type of food	Cal	Type of food	Cal
Bread, Light, 1slice	40	**Egg** Boiled, One	75	**Cantaloupe** 1 cup	55

Total calories 170

Type of food	Cal	Type of food	Cal
Hershey Almond Joy 1medium bar	180	**Sparkling water** 12 oz.	0

Total calories 180

Type of food	Cal	Type of food	Cal	Type of food	Cal
Arby's Scrambled eggs 2	140	**Grapefruit** ½ medium	40	**Coffee** No sweetener	1

Total calories 189

Breakfast

0-600 Calorie meals

Type of food **Denny's**	Cal	Type of food	Cal	Type of food	Cal
Chicken Noodle Soup 8 oz.	60	**Strawberries** 1 cup	50	**Melba toast** 4 pieces	80

Total calories 190

Type of food **Ham**, deli (4 avg. slices) 3 oz.	Cal	Type of food **Egg** Poached One	Cal	Type of food **Decaf Coffee** No sweetener	Cal
	120		75		1

Total calories 195

Type of food **Papa John's** Thin Crust Pizza Garden Special (large 14") 1/8, 124 g	Cal	Type of food **Diet coke** 12 oz.	Cal
	226		3

Total calories 229

Type of food **Oatmeal** 1 cup	Cal	Type of food **Banana** medium	Cal	Type of food **Sparkling water** 12 oz.	Cal
	150		115		0

Total calories 265

Type of food **Nestle –** 100 Grand 1 medium bar	Cal	Type of food **Raspberries** 1 cup	Cal	Type of food **Coffee** Artificial Sweetener	Cal
	200		60		3

Total calories 263

Breakfast

0-600 Calorie meals

Type of food	Cal	Type of food	Cal
Subway Western Egg or ham & egg (Breakfast Sandwich) 167 g	**290**	**Coffee** Artificial Sweetener	**3**

Total calories 293

Type of food	Cal	Type of food	Cal	Type of food	Cal
McDonald's Hash Browns 53 g	**130**	**McDonald's** Scrambled Eggs (2) 102 g	**160**	**Coffee** Artificial Sweetener	**3**

Total calories 293

Type of food	Cal	Type of food	Cal
McDonald's Egg McMuffin 138 g	**300**	**Decaf Coffee** No sweetener	**1**

Total calories 301

Type of food	Cal	Type of food	Cal	Type of food	Cal
1-Egg **sandwich** 1 regular dry	**225**	**Orange juice** 1 cup	**110**	**Coffee** Artificial Sweetener	**3**

Total calories 308

Type of food	Cal	Type of food	Cal	Type of food	Cal
McDonald's Lowfat Apple Bran Muffin 114 g	**300**	**Orange** 1 large	**80**	**Sparkling water** 12 oz.	**0**

Total calories 380

Breakfast

0-600 Calorie meals

Type of food	Cal	Type of food	Cal	Type of food	Cal
Bagel, Plain 1 Large (4 oz.)	300	**Banana** medium	115	**Coffee** Artificial Sweetener	3

Total calories 418

Type of food	Cal	Type of food	Cal	Type of food	Cal
Milk Whole 1pint	300	**English muffin** 1 medium	135	**Tea** Artificial Sweetener	3

Total calories 438

Type of food	Cal	Type of food	Cal	Type of food	Cal
Subway Cheese & Egg Breakfast Sandwich 130 g	302	**Orange juice** 1pt 16oz	220	**Coffee** Sweetener	33

Total calories 525

Type of food	Cal	Type of food	Cal	Type of food	Cal
Arby's Croissant with Bacon 76 g	340	**Arby's** Potato Cakes (2) 100 g	250	**Coffee** Artificial Sweetener	3

Total calories 593

R.L. Erickson C.H.P.

Snacks

Calories 0-300

Snacks
Calories 0-300

Type of food	Cal	Type of food	Cal
Celery, raw 1 stalk	5	**Cauliflower*** 1 cup	35
Carrots, raw 1 large	30	**Strawberries** 1 cup	50
Blackberries 1 cup	75	**Grapefruit** 1 medium	80
Apple 1 medium	80	**Corn on the cob*** 1 ear	80
Watermelon 1 pt.—16 oz.	100	**Banana** medium	115
Subway Peach Pizzazz Fuizie Express, small, 341 g	103	**Melba toast w/ Sour cream** 4 pieces	120
Kentucky Fried Chicken Original Recipe Chicken One whole wing	140	**Beer,** Generic 1 can, 12 oz.	145

Snacks
Calories 100-300

Type of food	Cal	*Type of food*	Cal
Pizza Hut thin'n crispy w /Ham medium pizza, 1 slice	170	*Cherry Cola* Sweetened 12 fl. oz.	180
Subway Oatmeal Raisin Cookie	197	**Kentucky Fried Chicken** Little Bucket Parfait Strawberry Shortcake	200
Apple 2 large	200	**Walnuts** ¼ cup	200
Candy bars 1 medium	170-280	**Cashews** 30	275

Lunch

Calories 100-500

Lunch
Calories 100-500

Type of food	Cal	Type of food	Cal	Type of food	Cal
Boston market Fruit salad, 6 oz.	**75**	**Apple** 1 medium	80	**Tea** Artificial Sweetener	3

Total Calories 158

Type of food	Cal	Type of food	Cal	Type of food	Cal
Spinach*, 1 cup	**40**	**Schlotzsky's** Minestrone Soup 227 g	89	**Saltines** 4 crackers	48

Total Calories 177

Type of food	Cal	Type of food	Cal	Type of food	Cal
Subway Roast Beef Salad 290 g	114	**Subway** Berry Lishus Fuizie Express small, 369 g	113	**Sparkling water** 12 oz.	0

Total Calories 227

Type of food	Cal	Type of food	Cal	Type of food	Cal
McDonald's Chef Salad 206 g	150	**McDonald's** Caesar Dressing 1 package, 44.4 ml	150	**Diet coke** caffeine-free	0

Total Calories 300

Type of food	Cal	Type of food	Cal	Type of food	Cal
Taco Bell Soft Taco – Chicken or Steak 3.5 oz.	190	**Taco Bell** Mexican Rice 4.75 oz.	190	**Diet coke** caffeine-free	0

Total Calories 380

Lunch
Calories 100-500

Type of food	Cal	Type of food	Cal	Type of food	Cal
Wendy's Crispy Chicken Nuggets (4 piece Kids' Meal) 60 g	190	**Wendy's** Deluxe Garden Salad 270 g	110	**Wendy's** Frosty Dairy Dessert Junior 113 g	170

Total Calories 470

Type of food	Cal	Type of food	Cal	Type of food	Cal
Arby's Grilled Chicken Salad 464 g	210	**Arby's** BBQ Vinaigrette Dressing 1 package, 2 oz.	140	*Ginger Ale* 12 fl. oz.	140

Total Calories 490

Type food	Cal	Type food	Cal	Type food	Cal
Tuna, Yellowfin, fresh (4x4x ¼") 6 oz.	240	**Mixed vegetables,** Frozen 1pint	220	**Peach** 1 medium	40

Total Calories 500

R.L. Erickson C.H.P.

Lunch

Calories 501-1000

Lunch
Calories 501-1000

Type of food	Cal	Type of food	Cal
		Wendy's	
Cola		Baked Potato	
Sweetened	**160**	Sour Cream & Chives	**370**
12 fl. oz.		312 g	

Total Calories 530

Type of food	Cal	Type of food	Cal	Type of food	Cal
Wendy's		**Wendy's**		**7-Up**	
Jr. Hamburger	**270**	Chili	**210**	Sweetened	**160**
117 g		small, 227 g		12 fl. oz	

Total Calories 640

Type of food	Cal	Type of food	Cal	Type of food	Cal
Taco Bell		**Taco Bell**			
2—Soft Taco	**520**	Cinnamon Twists	**150**	**Diet coke**	**0**
Supreme- Beef		1.25 oz.		caffeine-free	
10 oz.					

Total Calories 670

Type of food	Cal	Type of food	Cal	Type of food	Cal
Salmon,		**Mixed**			
Atlantic, fresh	**412**	**vegetables**,	**220**	**Strawberries**	**50**
½ lb.		Frozen		1 cup	
		1 pint			

Total Calories 682

Type of food	Cal	Type of food	Cal
Pizza Hut		*Cherry Cola*	
thin'n crispy w/Ham		Sweetened	**180**
medium pizza	**510**	12 fl. oz.	
3 slices, 246 g			

Total Calories 690

Lunch
Calories 701-1000

Type of food	Cal	Type of food	Cal	Type of food	Cal
Subway 6" Southwest Chicken 229 g	362	**Subway** Veggie Delite salad 3 oz.	60	**Milk** Whole 1 pint	300

Total Calories 722

Type of food	Cal	Type of food	Cal	Type of food	Cal
Burger King Chicken Whopper Jr. 165 g	350	**Burger King** Onion Rings - Large, 137 g	480	**Diet coke** caffeine-free	0

Total Calories 830

Type of food	Cal	Type of food	Cal
Kentucky Fried Chicken Hot & Spicy Chicken Breast 180 g	505	**Kentucky Fried Chicken** Little Bucket Parfait Lemon Crème 127g	410

Total Calories 915

Type of food	Cal	Type of food	Cal	Type of food	Cal
McDonald's Quarter Pounder 172 g	430	**McDonald's** Cinnamon Roll 95 g	390	**7-Up** Sweetened 12 fl. oz.	160

Total Calories 980

Type of food	Cal	Type of food	Cal
Pizza Hut Stuffed Crust veggie Lover's (medium pizza) 2 slices, 384 g	842	**Ginger Ale** 12 fl. oz.	140

Total Calories 982

R.L. Erickson C.H.P.

Dinner

Calories 301-700

Dinner
Calories 301-700

Type of food	Cal	Type of food	Cal	Type of food	Cal
Sweet potatoes or **yams,** baked 1 large, 8 oz.	230	**Oysters** 12 avg.	130	**Tea** Artificial Sweetener	3

Total Calories 363

Type of food	Cal	Type of food	Cal	Type of food	Cal
Wendy's Jr. Hamburger 117 g	270	**Zucchini** 1 cup	40	*Michelob* Light 1 can, 12 oz.	**135**

Total Calories 445

Type of food	Cal	Type of food	Cal	Type of food	Cal
Eggs Soufflé w/ Cheese 5 oz.	275	**Oatmeal** 1 cup	150	**Coffee** Artificial Sweetener	3

Total Calories 428

Type of food	Cal	Type of food	Cal	Type of food	Cal
Chicken breast, no skin 1large- 5 oz.	233	**Refried beans,** Fat-free 1 cup	220	**Burgundy,** White 1 glass, 4 fl. oz.	90

Total Calories 543

Type of food	Cal	Type of food	Cal	Type of food	Cal
T-bone or Porterhouse steak ¼ lb.	340	*Rice* White, 1 cup	260	**Tea** Artificial Sweetener	3

Total Calories 603

Dinner
Calories 301-700

Type of food	Cal	Type of food	Cal	Type of food	Cal	Type of food	Cal
Crab, blue, fresh 1 lb.	480	**Carrots,** raw 1 large	30	**Artichoke** 1 medium	60	**Champagne,** dry 1 glass, 4 oz.	105

Total Calories 675

Type of food	Cal	Type of food	Cal	Type of food	Cal
Pork tenderloin 8 oz.	372	**Potato,** baked w/butter 1large, 8 oz	325	**Coffee** artificial sweetener	3

Total Calories 700

R.L. Erickson C.H.P.

Dinner

Calories 701-1100

Dinner
Calories 701-1100

Type of food	Cal	Type of food	Cal	Type of food	Cal
Sausage, Italian ¼ lb.	430	**Cabbage*** 2cups	60	**Dry beans**, Cooked 1cup	240

Total Calories 730

Type of food	Cal	Type of food	Cal	*Type of food*	Cal
Burger King BK Veggie Burger 173 g	330	**Burger King** Dutch Apple Pie 113 g	340	*Lemon-Lime* 12 fl. oz.	140

Total Calories 810

Type of food	Cal
Denny's Classic Burger with Cheese	836

Total Calories 836

Type of food	Cal	Type of food	Cal	Type of food	Cal
Wendy's Blue Cheese Dressing 1 packet, 57 g	360	**Wendy's** Deluxe Garden Salad 270 g	110	**Wendy's** Jr. Hamburger 117 g	270

Total Calories 840

Type of food	Cal	Type of food	Cal	Type of food	Cal
McDonald's French Fries Small 68 g	210	**McDonald's** Hot Caramel Sundae 182 g	360	**McDonald's** Chicken McNuggets 6 pieces, 108 g	310

Total Calories 880

Dinner
Calories 701-1100

Ham
8 oz.　　**359**

Cheese,
Reduced fat
4 oz.　　**360**

Cabernet
Sauvignon
2 glasses,
8 fl. oz.　　**180**

Total Calories 899

Burger King
Double Whopper
(w/o Mayo) 380 g　　**900**

Total Calories 900

Artichoke Hearts
Marinated
1 cup

220

Turkey,
Light meat and
skin, roasted
10 oz.

642

Blackberries　**75**
1 cup

Total Calories 937

Hardees
Monster Burger
288 g　　**1,060**

Total Calories 1060

Rib Eye,
fat, broiled
8 oz.

657

Cottage
cheese
(2%)
1 cup

200

Potatoes mashed
With milk and
butter
1 cup

220

Total Calories 1077

Table 1. Food energy and macronutrients per capita per day in the U.S. food supply by decade, 1909-99*

	Carbohydrate	fiber	Protein	fat
Kilocalories				
1909-19 3400	486	28	96	120
1920-29 3400	474	26	92	127
1930-39 3300	447	25	89	129
1940-49 3300	426	24	98	138
1950-59 3100	386	20	93	138
1960-69 3100	379	18	93	143
1970-79 3200	387	19	95	149
1980-89 3400	411	20	98	156
1990-99 3700	478	23	108	159

Gerrior, S. and Bente,, L. 2002. *Nutrient Content of the U.S. Food Supply, 1909-99: A Summary Report.* U.S. Department of Agriculture, Center for Nutrition Policy and Promotion. Home Economics Research Report No. 55.

Weekly Worksheet

Week # _____ **Date (mo./day)** _____ **to** _____

Starting weight _____ **Goal weight** _____

Measurements: arms ___ neck___ chest___ waist___ hips___
calves ___

Base Number_____Activity Level- Inactive __ Average __ Active __

Daily Step Rate Max.

DAY	Allotted Calories	Calories consumed	Over/under
ONE	_____	_____	_____
TWO	_____	_____	_____
THREE	_____	_____	_____
FOUR	_____	_____	_____
FIVE	_____	_____	_____
SIX	_____	_____	_____
SEVEN	_____	_____	_____
Totals	_____	_____	_____ *

- NOTE: If you are within 200 calories of your total weekly calorie maximum and you did not lose weight, drop back one space on your base number. Example;(**Base number 8 –average—** drops back to **Base number 8 –inactive—** on your daily calorie maximums).

Favorite foods chart

List your favorite foods below for easy reference

Food	nutritional value:	good	junk
1. _____		____	____
2. _____		____	____
3. _____		____	____
4. _____		____	____
5. _____		____	____
6. _____		____	____
7. _____		____	____
8. _____		____	____
9. _____		____	____
10. _____		____	____
11. _____		____	____
12. _____		____	____
13. _____		____	____
14. _____		____	____
15. _____		____	____
16. _____		____	____
17. _____		____	____

<u>NOTES</u>

<u>NOTES</u>

Suggested readings

A User's Guide tTo The Brain. John J. Ratey, M.D. Random house New York 2001

Clinical and Experimental Hypnosis. 2ND Edition William S. Kroger, M.D. J.B. Lippincott Company Philadelphia, Pennsylvania 1977

Visualization and Guided Imagery for Pain Management. R.D. Longacre, PH.D. Kendall/Hunt Publishing Company Dubuque, Iowa 1995

The Owners Manual for The Brain. 2ND Edition Pierce J. Howard, PH.D. Bard Press Marietta GA.2000

Toward a Science of Consciousness. Stuart R. Hameroff M.D. MIT press Cambridge Massachusetts 1996

The Nature of Emotion. Robert Ekman and Richard Davidson. Oxford University Press, New York 1994

Phantoms in the Brain. V.S. Ramachandran, M.D. and Sandra Blakeslee. William Morrow, New York, 1998

Your Emotions and Your Heath. Emrika Padus. Rodale Press, Emmaus Pennsylvania 1986

Know your fats. Mary G. Enig PH.D. Bethesda Press, 2000

The Cholesterol Myths. Uffe Ravnskov M.D. PH.D. New Trends Publishing Inc. Winona Lake, IN 2000

The Homocysteine Revolution. Kilmer S. McCully M.D. McGraw/Hill Contemporary books 1999

The Relaxation Response. Herbert Benson, M.D. HarperCollins Publishers New York 2000

The World Book. World Book Encyclopedia, World Book Inc., 2001

Internet web sites of interest

Mental Image
http://salve.slam.katowice.pl/equi-me-rec-unit.htm

Saturated fats and the kidneys
http://www.westonaprice.org/know_your_fats/kidneys_fats.html

How stuff works fats
http://www.westonaprice.org/know_your_fats/kidneys_fats.html

Neurotransmitters for kids
http://faculty.washington.edu/chudler/chnt1.html

Human body experience –muscle
http://vilenski.org/science/humanbody/hb_html/muscles.html

USDA Nutrient Data Base
http://www.nal.usda.gov/fnic/foodcomp/

Meals.com –nutrition
http://www.my-meals.com/FeaturesAndAdvice/Nutrition.aspx?Menu=16

CNN: Health genes that alter fat storage
http://www.cnn.com/2000/HEALTH/diet.fitness/11/14/thrifty.gene.ap/

LIFE –Enhancement caloric restriction
http://www.life-enhancement.com/displayart.asp?ID=532

LIFE EXTENTION-Our Big Fat Problem
http://www.lef.org/newsarchive/nutrition/2001/06/10/F/32923717-0030-Home.html

Brain Evolution
http://brainmuseum.org/Evolution/

Closer to the Truth
http://www.closertotruth.com/

The Limbic System
http://www.epub.org.br/cm/n05/mente/limbic_i.htm

Human Digestion
http://www.borg.com/~lubehawk/hdigsys.htm

Internet web sites of interest

The Hippocratic Oath
http://members.tripod.com/adm/popup/roadmap.shtml?member_name=nktiu
ro&path=hippocra.htm&client_ip=152.163.188.199&ts=1035134331&ad_typ
e=POPUP&id=ae90e5ccabf06eacdf81c685eb273c4d

What is Ockham's Razor?
http://phyun5.ucr.edu/~wudka/Physics7/Notes_www/node10.html#SECTION
02125000000000000000

Introduction to the Scientific Method
http://teacher.nsrl.rochester.edu/phy_labs/AppendixE/AppendixE.html#Head
ing3

How a New Policy Led to Seven Deadly Drugs
http://www.msbp.com/fda.htm

Exercise Myths
http://www.womans-work.com/Life_Balance/Exercise_Myths.htm

Types of neurons
http://faculty.washington.edu/chudler/cells.html

Prescription Medication for the Treatment of Obesity
http://www.niddk.nih.gov/health/nutrit/pubs/presmeds.htm#meds

U.S. Food Supply Providing More Food and Calories
http://www.ers.usda.gov/publications/foodreview/sep1999/frsept99a.pdf

Food supply 1909-1999
http://www.usda.gov/cnpp/Pubs/Food%20Supply/foodsupply09_99.pdf

Good side to cholesterol?
http://www.goodnewscholesterol.com/

Nutrition and Metabolism
file:///C:/WINDOWS/Temporary%20Internet%20Files/Content.IE5/SHAZ416
Z/nutritionmetabolism%5B1%5D.ppt#256,1,%20Nutrition%20and%20Metab
olism

Energy in foods
http://www.healthyeatingclub.com/info/books-
phds/books/foodfacts/html/data/data2a.html

Internet web sites of interest

Consumption
http://www.mindfully.org/Sustainability/Consumption-Industrialized-Commercialized.htm

Population
http://bioweb.wku.edu/courses/BIOL115/Wyatt/Population/pop1.htm

Foods Sold in Competition with USDA School Meal Programs
http://www.fns.usda.gov/cnd/Lunch/CompetitveFoods/competitive.foods.report.to.congress.htm

Calories and fats alphabetically
http://www.ntwrks.com/~mikev/chart1.html

The Metabolism Myth
http://www.cbass.com/METABOLI.HTM

Sneaky serving sizes
http://www.fourmilab.ch/hackdiet/www/subsubsection1_3_2_0_6_2.html

Basal Metabolic Rate (BMR
http://instruct1.cit.cornell.edu/Courses/ns421/BMR.html

Fat-Free vs. Regular Calorie Comparison
http://www.fda.gov/fdac/features/2002/chrt_calcomp.html

Hypothalamus and ANS
http://thalamus.wustl.edu/course/hypoANS.html

History of Agriculture
http://www.crystalinks.com/agriculturehistory2.html

Physical Activity Fundamental To Preventing Disease
http://aspe.hhs.gov/health/reports/physicalactivity/

Evolution, Diet and Health
http://www.cast.uark.edu/local/icaes/conferences/wburg/posters/sboydeaton/eaton.htm

Contact information

Reducing stress is the main key to losing excess stored body fat. Mr. Erickson's relaxation weight loss audio CD has been especially designed for those with Habitual Eating Syndrome. You may purchase the relaxation CD and additional authored materials by Mr. Erickson from our web site at

www.RLErickson.org

Or by calling 1-800-449-0146

Coming in April 2003

<u>Habitual Smoking Syndrome</u>

Are you or someone you know smoking? An estimated 8 out of 10 smokes are "habit smokers" that don't know how to stop. My new book will help the "habit smokers" become non-smoker Mr. Erickson has a private practice in Carmel In. He can be contacted via his web sites. He is available for personal counseling, small group sessions, lectures, seminars, and book signings.

www.thehypnotist.net

If you would like to be a distributor of Mr. Erickson's works please contact us at 1-800-449-0146

R.L. Erickson C.H.P.

About the Author

At age nine, Richard L. Erickson sustained a head trauma after being struck by a motorist, which was the precursor to Grand Mal Epileptic seizure activity that lasted into his forties. The resolve to "*Never give up.*" was also a by-product of that event.

In his teens, he was laughed at and ridiculed because of epileptic seizures, denied an auto license, rejected by the armed services, and not allowed to play certain college sports. After receiving his Bachelor of Science degree from Ball State University, he spent many years in marketing.

At age thirty-seven he was diagnosed with coronary heart disease and advised to exercise. His resolve took him one step farther. Realizing the importance of fitness, nutrition, and the minds effects on the body, at age 40 Mr. Erickson, along with his wife Susan, founded Motivations Fitness Centers Inc, and in 1991 he began to study the mind-body relationship through the science of hypnosis. This lead to setting six world weightlifting records, placing fifth, in his class, in the Mr. America bodybuilding championships and became a nationally recognized personal trainer.

Today Mr. Erickson is an author, leading Indiana Hypnotist practitioner, owner of The Carmel Hypnosis Center and two health clubs, a world-class weight lifting champion, nationally certified personal trainer, and motivational public speaker. He is committed to helping people overcome the misinformation and obstacles laid in the path of life for the deconditioned, and mentally and emotionally challenged.

Mr. Erickson is available for book signings, large and small lectures, motivational speeches, and one-on-one hypnosis sessions. You may reach him by writing, calling, e-mailing or faxing his Carmel office.

The Carmel Hypnosis Center

820 West 122nd St.

Carmel In. 46032

1-800-449-0146

(317) 843-0683

Fax 317-580-8116

www.rlerickson.org

Printed in the United States
1396900003B/52-222